The PRITIKIN EDGE

10 Essential Ingredients for a Long and Delicious Life

Dr. Robert A. Vogel and Paul Tager Lehr

Food plans by Eugenia Killoran
With photographs by Michael Fryd

SIMON & SCHUSTER
New York • London • Toronto • Sydney

This publication contains the opinions and ideas of its authors. It is intended to provide helpful and informative material on the subjects addressed in the publication. It is sold with the understanding that the authors and publisher are not engaged in rendering medical, health, psychological, or any other kind of personal professional services in the book. If the reader requires personal medical, health, or other assistance or advice, a competent professional should be consulted.

The authors and publisher specifically disclaim all responsibility for any liability, loss, or risk, personal or otherwise, that is incurred as a consequence, directly or indirectly, of the use and application of any of the contents of this book.

Before starting on a weight-loss plan, or beginning or modifying an exercise program, check with your physician to make sure that the changes are right for you.

Simon & Schuster
1230 Avenue of the Americas
New York, NY 10020

Copyright © 2008 by Dr. Robert Vogel and The Pritikin Organization, LLC
Photographs copyright © 2008 by Michael Fryd

All rights reserved, including the right to reproduce this book or portions thereof in any form whatsoever. For information address Simon & Schuster Subsidiary Rights Department, 1230 Avenue of the Americas, New York, NY 10020

First Simon & Schuster hardcover edition September 2008

SIMON & SCHUSTER and colophon are registered trademarks of Simon & Schuster, Inc.

For information about special discounts for bulk purchases, please contact Simon & Schuster Special Sales at 1-800-456-6789 or business@simonandschuster.com.

Designed by Dana Sloan

Manufactured in the United States of America

10   9   8   7   6   5   4   3   2   1

Library of Congress Cataloging-in-Publication Data

Vogel, Robert A., 1943–
The Pritikin edge / Robert A. Vogel & Paul Tager Lehr.
p.   cm.
1. Low-fat diet.   2. Health.   3. Pritikin, Nathan.   4. Coronary heart disease—Diet therapy.   I. Lehr, Paul Tager.   II. Title.
RM237.7.V64 2008
613.2'5—dc22   2008015285

ISBN-13: 978-1-4165-8088-1
ISBN-10:   1-4165-8088-3

Dedicated to my wife and domestic goddess, Sharyn Lynn, who has given me many lessons in living deliciously and the reason for living long; my daughter and her family, Elizabeth Ann, Robert Elias, Delaney Grace, Charlotte Elizabeth, and Jasper Elias, who overflow with emotional nourishment; the Pritikin faculty, who share the same vision of living well; Drs. Bruce Paton and William Oetgen, who tried to make sense of my scribbles; and my patients, who have taught me so much more than I taught them.

—*Bob Vogel*

Dedicated to David Lehr, M.D., my father and inspiration, and without whom the Pritikin Program would never have gotten off the ground; to Mira Lehr, my rock and brilliant-artist mother; my nearly perfect wife Jeannine (ask anybody); and my sweet and wonderful children, David and Tager, who give greater meaning to my life; and my siblings (also sweet and wonderful) Alison, John, and Elizabeth. Special thanks and appreciation to my mentor and surrogate father Ambassador Sam Fox and Marilyn Fox, whose unending faith in me and passion for Pritikin mean more than they know and will help keep me alive for a long time and Pritikin alive forever, and to Dr. Bauer and all of the inspiring people on the Pritikin team with whom I have worked for years and who make the Pritikin Program truly exceptional.

—*Paul Lehr*

Acknowledgments

WE WISH TO thank Debra Goldstein, who helped us capture the essence of the Pritikin Program.

And, of course, special thanks to all of the 100,000 plus people who have attended the residential programs at the Pritikin Longevity Center and Spa, and the 10 million readers who have followed our advice and helped us learn and grow and allowed us to continue Pritikin's mission to wipe obesity, heart disease, and other lifestyle diseases from the face of the earth.

Contents

Foreword

SOMETHING MADE YOU buy this book. What was it? A medical scare? A stern warning from your doctor about your high cholesterol or blood pressure? Excess weight? Chest pain—better known as your body's final announcement that you should lay off the double cheeseburgers?

Ultimately, it doesn't really matter. What matters is that by picking up this book, you're already on your way to a better life, one in which health of body and mind are not only possible, but absolutely achievable.

We Americans may reside in the greatest nation on Earth, but we actually live a third-world lifestyle. One-quarter of us still smoke, two-thirds of us are fat, three-quarters of us don't exercise, and stress and depression are ubiquitous. We wolf down humongous portions of fast food in minutes, boast of not taking a vacation in years, and have the communal longevity of a banana republic. On the surface, we are strong and productive. Underneath, our lifestyle is killing us, lead primarily by an epidemic of heart disease. Heart disease claims as many lives in America every day as the 9/11 disaster did once. It's time for us to wake up and start making changes: not just in what we eat, but in how we live.

The Pritikin Program was the first comprehensive lifestyle program in America. After 50 years on the cutting edge of lifestyle science, Pritikin is still the longest-running, most successful program for reversing many of modern society's diseases, including obesity, heart disease, and diabetes. What sets Pritikin apart from the myriad of Johnny-come-lately diets is that its program is based on *real science.* It employs the three-step scientific process of observation, theories, and proof: observations on how thin, healthy people live; theories about why healthy practices work; and confirmation in scientific trials that our recommendations actually work. We don't make random claims or base our advice on half-truths or fads; we base our knowledge on research that has, over the past three decades, been confirmed in more than 110 scientific studies.

My first trip to the Pritikin Longevity Center was eye-opening for me. In the world of medicine, I am known as the lifestyle cardiologist. Like Nathan Pritikin, I believe in making changes from the inside out, rather than relying on medications or passing trends. In treating my patients, I focus on the whole person: what and how much they eat, how much exercise they get, and how they manage stress and other emotional issues. When I experienced the program at Pritikin, I was thrilled: here was an entire program whose practices and principles were nearly identical to mine! I felt right at home, from the healthy food they offer to their fascinating curriculum of lifestyle lectures on everything from stress reduction to nutrition to how to decipher the ridiculously confusing language on food labels. Their nutritional philosophy was smart—no "glycemic index" nonsense, no "olive oil is healthy" rhetoric (it isn't, but I'll get to that later on). I arrived there thinking I knew everything there was to know about lifestyle health, but, boy, was I mistaken! It turns out there was still plenty for this cardiologist to learn. I became more and more involved with the Pritikin Center, and in 2007, I was appointed their chief medical director.

In this book, you will learn the real truth about heart disease, obesity, weight loss, and why lifestyle changes are the key to living a healthy, happy life. We will share with you the 10 essential ingredients of the Pritikin Program, which deal with diet, exercise, and overall emotional wellness. The 10 essentials are the foundation of the Pritikin philosophy, and have changed the lives of hundreds of thousands of people world-wide.

Altering just one aspect of your lifestyle might make a small dent, but if you're looking for sustainable health practices that will give back to you *seven years* of happy, healthy living, it's time for a sweeping systemic change. I promise, once you get started living these principles, you'll wonder how or why you ever lived any other way. You'll lose weight without feeling hungry, regain your vitality, and look and feel healthier, stronger, and more vibrant—more *alive.* The days of excess weight and potential heart disease will be behind you. Now's your chance.

Dr. Robert Vogel
February 2008

Introduction

I CANNOT REMEMBER a time when the Pritikin Program was not a part of my life. As a 10-year-old in 1977, I watched my father, cardiologist David Lehr, M.D., appear with Nathan Pritikin on *60 Minutes* and introduce to America an entirely new approach to the treatment of heart disease. Passionately and compellingly, my dad argued that Americans should turn to daily exercise and a low-fat, high-fiber diet full of whole foods like fruits, vegetables, and whole grains. At the time, his words were revolutionary. They were also courageous. He had defied the medical establishment of which he was a part. Today, the medical profession and the American Heart Association recommend this lifestyle approach as the first line of defense against coronary artery disease.

The Pritikin Program—and the search for a better American lifestyle—began 50 years ago when Nathan Pritikin, age 41, was diagnosed with heart disease. Doctors from UCLA told Nathan he should take it easy (lot of naps and no exercise) and keep eating his usual diet, full of butter, ice cream, and steaks.

But the inventor and engineer started doing his own research. Studying countries around the world, Nathan realized that populations consuming a lot of saturated fat-rich red meat and dairy foods had the highest rates of heart disease. By contrast, populations eating less saturated fat and more unrefined, unprocessed whole foods rarely suffered heart attacks. These heart-healthy populations also exercised daily. Their cholesterol levels rarely exceeded 160.

Nathan's own cholesterol was 280, a value considered normal at that time—the late 1950s. His doctors emphatically warned him that if he started exercising and fooling around with his diet, he might kill himself. Frightened but determined, he traded his butter, ice cream, and steak diet for one rich in fruits, vegetables, whole grains, and beans. He also started walking, then jogging, three to five miles daily. His cholesterol plummeted to 120. Two years later, an electrocardiogram showed no evidence of heart disease.

Emboldened by Nathan's new life, the Pritikin team launched dozens of research projects over the next five decades. Study after study validated the many benefits of the Pritikin Program, which recommends daily exercise and a diet naturally low in fat, emphasizing fruits, vegetables, whole grains, beans, lean meat, seafood, and nonfat dairy products. To date, more than 110 scientific studies have been published in leading medical publications proving the efficacy of the *therapeutic* Pritikin Program, which has been followed by more than 100,000 people at the Pritikin Longevity Center. For the complete bibliography, I invite you to visit www.pritikin.com. Below are highlights. Within three to four weeks, the Pritikin Program has been proven to do the following.

Markedly Reduce Key Risk Factors for Heart Disease

- *Cholesterol*: Analyses of 4,587 guests staying at Pritikin for three weeks showed an average 23 percent drop in total cholesterol and 23 percent drop in LDL bad cholesterol. *Archives of Internal Medicine* 151: 1389, 1991.
- *Triglycerides*: These 4,587 Pritikin guests also reduced triglycerides on average 33 percent. *Archives of Internal Medicine* 151: 1389, 1991.

- *C-Reactive Protein*: In just two weeks, inflammation markers like C-reactive protein plunged 45 percent in women at the Pritikin Center. No other lifestyle-change program or drug therapy, including statins, has proven to lower C-reactive protein so dramatically or rapidly. *Metabolism* 53: 377, 2004.

Substantially Enhance the Effectiveness of Statin Therapy/Reduce Statin Need

Prior to attending Pritikin, 93 men and women had reduced their total and LDL cholesterol levels about 20 percent on statins. After two weeks at Pritikin, they demonstrated an additional 19 percent decrease in cholesterol levels. *American Journal of Cardiology* 79: 1112, 1997.

Lower Blood Pressure to Normal, Medication-Free Levels

In a study of 268 men, 83 percent lowered their blood pressure to normal levels and left free of all drugs for hypertension. *Journal of Cardiac Rehabilitation* 3: 839, 1983. See also *Circulation* 106: 2530, 2002. In a meta-analysis of 1,117 hypertensives, 55 percent normalized blood pressure and no longer required medications within three weeks of starting the Pritikin Program. *Journal of Applied Physiology* 98: 3, 2005.

Control Diabetes and, for Many, Eliminate the Need for Drugs

A meta analysis of 864 type 2 diabetics found that 74 percent on oral agents left Pritikin free of such medications, their blood sugars in normal ranges, and 44 percent on insulin left insulin-free. Those who continued the Pritikin Program stayed off the medications. *Journal of Applied Physiology* 98: 3, 2005. See also *Diabetes Care* 17: 1469, 1994.

Reverse the Metabolic Syndrome

Having the metabolic syndrome, a condition now epidemic in the U.S., puts one at major risk for diabetes and heart disease. In about 50 percent of men studied, the Pritikin Program reversed the clinical diagnosis of metabolic syndrome. *Journal of Applied Physiology* 100: 1657, 2006.

Eliminate the Need for Angioplasty and Bypass Surgery; Relieve Angina Pain

A five-year study of 64 men who came to Pritikin instead of undergoing the recommended bypass surgery found that 80 percent never needed the surgery. Of those taking drugs for angina (chest) pain, 62 percent left the Center pain-free and drug-free. *Journal of Cardiac Rehabilitation* 3: 183, 1983.

Promote Healthy Weight Loss

Men and women needing to lose weight lost on average 10 pounds within three weeks of starting the Pritikin Program. *Archives of Internal Medicine* 151: 1389, 1991.

Reduce Key Risk Factors for Breast, Colon, and Prostate Cancer

Groundbreaking studies showed that the Pritikin Program retarded the growth of both breast cancer and prostate cancer cells in laboratory testing, and even induced tumor cells to self-destruct. *Cancer Causes and Control* 13: 929, 2002; *Nutrition and Cancer* 55 (1): 28, 2006.

In addition to all of Pritikin's scientific investigations, Nathan Pritikin himself benefited greatly from his program. When he died in 1985 after a decades-long fight with leukemia, the autopsy report, published in the *New England Journal of Medicine,* showed that he had actually reversed the heart disease and plaque buildup he had been diagnosed with which had inspired the program. It was written that his arteries were "soft and pliable" and that "the near absence of atherosclerosis and the complete absence of its effects are remarkable."

Today at the Pritikin Longevity Center, I'm proud to say that I continue the work of my father and Nathan Pritikin. I lead a world-class research institution that continues to investigate healthful living, part of the nonprofit Pritikin Foundation. I also lead a faculty of nationally acclaimed physicians, registered dietitians, psychologists, and exercise physiologists who teach thousands of guests annually the Pritikin Program, helping them not only lose weight permanently but also live longer, healthier, and more active lives. I can't imagine a better job!

With more than 30 years of clinical experience, the Pritikin Center has helped more than 100,000 people regain their health and vitality with its life-enhancing *therapeutic* program. *The Pritikin Edge,* written by Dr. Robert Vogel, our chief medical director, and myself, and with the help of all our faculty at Pritikin, draws on our thirty years of experience and gives you the tools you need to look better, feel better—and best of all, live better.

Paul Lehr
President, Pritikin Longevity Center & Spa
February 2008

PART ONE

The Pritikin
Philosophy

1

Lifestyle and Heart Disease

YOU KNOW BILL. At 58 years old, a strapping six feet two inches tall and 220 pounds with a full head of silver hair, he was outwardly the picture of power and health. He received great medical care. He jogged and golfed frequently. But just like most Americans, Bill loved food—especially fatty, spicy, salty food. His typical American extra pounds pushed his blood pressure, sugar, and LDL (bad) cholesterol too high and dropped his HDL (good) cholesterol too low. He lived with chronic stress, big time. None of his numbers were awful, but every warning sign was there.

One day Bill had chest pain. The next week, his quadruple coronary bypass was all over the news, because Bill is President Bill Clinton. Yes, even American presidents can get heart disease. Since his wake-up call, Mr. Clinton has changed his lifestyle quite a bit. He is now off the ribs and fries and is working hard to do his part to prevent heart disease in this country.

Improving your lifestyle after a heart attack or bypass surgery is certainly a step in the right direction, but wouldn't it be so much better to do so *before* you end up in the coronary care unit or surgical suite? Or worse, the morgue? Our guests at the Pritikin Longevity Center sometimes complain that they don't have enough time to exercise. We remind them that they will have plenty of time to exercise, but not much inclination after they are dead.

Heart disease is a great barometer of a lousy lifestyle. Wherever heart disease is epidemic, so are obesity, high blood pressure, high cholesterol, stroke, and diabetes. Obviously, few people are heeding the early warning signs, because I don't know any fellow cardiologists looking for more work. We live in fear of cancer, but heart disease is still the number-one killer in America. I wish I could tell you how to avoid most cancers. Sadly, I can't. But I can tell you how to prevent most heart disease simply by changing your lifestyle. Some cancers may even be avoided by these same lifestyle changes. What you eat, how often you exercise, how you manage your stress . . . it all matters, and it's all easier to improve than you might think.

THE 10 ESSENTIAL INGREDIENTS OF THE PRITIKIN PROGRAM

In this book, you will learn the 10 essential ingredients of the Pritikin Program. These 10 Pritikin essentials deal with diet, exercise, and emotional wellness. By adopting these lifestyle practices, as thousands of our patients and participants have, you will get back the *seven years* of life you might otherwise lose to heart disease. (By the way, if seven years doesn't seem important to you right now, imagine how much more important they will seem to you when you're 75.) You will learn how to lose weight permanently without feeling hungry, to cook really tasty, heart-healthy food, the best ways to be physically active, and how to sidestep stress. You will learn the real science of lifestyle and heart health, so that you are able to make choices every single day that will contribute to your wellness and enable you to live a long, delicious life.

You'll learn much more in Part Two about the specifics of the 10 essential ingredients of the Pritikin Program, but here is a quick glance:

1. Healthy, satisfying eating starts with super salads, soups, whole grains, and fruit.
2. Eliminate high-calorie beverages.
3. Trim portions of calorie-dense foods.
4. Snack smarter.
5. Forget fast food; dine unrefined.
6. Watch less, walk more.
7. Go lean on meat, but catch a fish.
8. Shake your salt habit.
9. Don't smoke your life away.
10. Step around stress.

Adopting one or two of these essential lifestyle practices is okay, but *optimal health requires that you follow the whole program.* Why? Because obesity, inactivity, heart disease, and emotions are intricately connected. Couch potatoes tend to be depressed; depressed people eat more; people who eat more gain weight; those who gain weight tend to sack out on the couch rather than exercise; lack of exercise contributes to heart disease; heart disease can trigger depression . . . you get the picture. You may already be following several lifestyle essentials, but now is your chance to complete the program and get all seven years back, not to mention being able to more fully enjoy your life right here and now.

THE PRITIKIN PHILOSOPHY

The Pritikin Program is simple, thorough, and most of all, smart. No gimmicks, fads, pseudo-science, or rhetoric here. The philosophy is based on five main points:

- Heart disease is best prevented through lifestyle changes.
- Emotional wellness and heart healthiness are intricately connected.
- Wellness is much more than the absence of illness.
- Complex health problems do not have simple solutions.
- Illness and wellness are global issues: they affect families, communities, and nations.

Lifestyle Changes versus Medication

I love sushi. Almost every day while we had a sushi bar in our hospital, I would eat ahi along with a green salad. One day, without notice, the sushi bar disappeared; it seems it wasn't making the hospital money. After all, why lose money selling tasty food that just might prevent heart disease when you can get paid a great deal to treat it? Sayonara, sushi bar. Did I complain? You bet! Now it's back.

This story illustrates the paradox of our unhealthy culture and medical care. When we become ill, we immediately turn to drugs to fix the consequences of a poor lifestyle. We focus on fixing a problem after we've created it, rather than trying to prevent it altogether.

Pop a pill, or hop on the treadmill—which is easier? Taking a pill, of course. Which is better? Hands down, preventing the illness that mandates the pill in the first place through healthy living. When we change our lifestyle, we not only negate the need for costly medications, we lessen our risk of developing a myriad of diseases, including diabetes, cancer, arthritis, and depression, not to mention heart disease, because these common afflictions share many of the same root causes.

I readily admit I will use medications in my practice to lower cholesterol in patients who will not change their lifestyle or for whom this change is not enough. But time and again, I've seen that my patients who do lower their cholesterol through diet and exercise rather than medication look and feel better. Yes, they have to put in a little more time and effort than it takes to pry the top off a pill bottle, but the quality of their lives is far superior. They are more physically fit, emotionally engaged, and energized by their ability to improve their well-being.

Prescriptions or Power Walks? Consider This:

- Most lifestyle changes are free, or very inexpensive. Salads are still cheaper than any prescription drug.
- You don't need preapproval from an HMO to go for a long walk.
- Lifestyle changes have few negative side effects. You don't have to worry about mixing good habits, and I have never had a patient allergic to walking.
- The most valuable lifestyle changes have no drug substitutes. As yet, we have not been able to capture all the benefits of friendship and love in a pill.

Emotions and Heart Disease

Our metaphorical "heart," from which we feel love and affection, and our physical heart are actually one and the same. How you feel can absolutely affect your cardiovascular health. As we like to say at Pritikin, a happy life equals a happy heart.

Depressed people tend to eat poorly, smoke more frequently, and exercise rarely—all major contributors to heart disease. There is a lot of research that shows depression and anger increase the chronic factors that contribute to heart disease, most specifically inflammation and a decrease in protective chemicals like nitric oxide (more on this in Chapter 2). And, not surprisingly, the relationship works both ways: depression and anger frequently follow heart attacks and bypass surgery.

Can you die of a broken heart? Absolutely. Faced with sudden emotional stress, your heart can actually stop pumping effectively. Learning about the death or illness of a loved one can do it; this is literally called "broken heart syndrome." In response to extreme stress or grief, an outpour of adrenaline and related hormones can stun the heart, mimicking a heart attack.

Fortunately, though, the same holds true in reverse. Upbeat emotions and heart healthiness are also intricately connected. It has been proven that watching 30 minutes of a humorous video relaxes your blood vessels. Socially and spiritually connected people, such as churchgoers and others who are socially active, tend to live healthier lifestyles and thus experience less heart disease. In one of the best-known studies of cardiac health, the Normative Aging Study done in VA hospitals, it was shown that optimistic men actually have few heart attacks.

There's another component to the link between emotions and heart health: think about how your self-image improves with weight loss and the joy of shopping for slimmer clothes. I know of few compliments more welcome in our society than being told that you look like you lost weight. (By the way, I've come to learn that the only correct answer to your wife's question of whether a dress makes her look fat is, "How could it, dear?")

Wellness versus Absence of Illness

Just like illness, health and wellness come in degrees. You may not be ill, but can you run a 6-minute mile—or even a 12-minute mile? You may not be depressed, but are you truly happy? You may not have had a heart attack or stroke yet, but do you really think that all those double cheeseburgers and French fries have not done you any damage?

We call heart disease the silent killer. You usually feel fine the day before a heart attack or stroke, but you are really a coronary time bomb. Did you know that 85 percent of 50-year-old people have blockage in the arteries of their hearts without any symptoms? It is a tragedy that high blood pressure and cholesterol aren't painful until it is too late.

True wellness is not just the absence of known disease, but also the promise that you will remain well for some time to come. By following the 10 essential ingredients in the Pritikin Program, you are laying the foundation for a lifetime of health.

No Simple Solutions

I have a real bee in my bonnet about quick-fix promises to health or weight loss. Most of them, to be perfectly frank, are hogwash. There are no simple solutions to complex issues of health and lifestyle. Healthy eating cannot be summarized in single sound bites, like "avoid carbs" or "drink red wine." If it were that simple, we'd all be fit and healthy at the snap of our fingers.

Maybe you're thinking of trying a low-carb/high-protein (and thus usually high-fat) diet to lose weight. The truth is that some fats in excess cause heart disease. A skinny waistline is great, but not at the risk of a heart attack or stroke.

Drinking a little alcohol regularly does reduce some heart problems, that's true. But too much alcohol weakens the heart and causes high blood pressure and irregular heartbeats.

We don't offer quick-fix solutions at Pritikin, because we know better. We know that fads (low-carb), half-truths ("olive oil is good for you"), and popular impressions (anything "natural" must be healthy) are all tempting in their simplicity, but ultimately misleading.

Heart Disease Is a Community Concern

We share our physical and emotional health with everyone around us. Think about it: if you cook unhealthy food or take your family to fast-food restaurants, you are propagating obesity, diabetes, and heart disease. If you smoke, you are turning the people around you into secondhand smokers, and your children are more likely to follow you down that deadly road and become smokers themselves. If you drive five blocks to a store instead of walking, you are adding to our already clogged roads and overflowing parking lots and polluting our already smog-filled air. Your lost days of work due to illness put a strain on your coworkers and company (not to mention your wallet).

As great as this country is, we have too much obesity and physical inactivity, too many workaholics, and too few people living joyously.

If our typical fast food were really delicious and nutritious, I could better tolerate the obesity. If we had great longevity, I could better tolerate the inactivity. If we were broadly happy, I could better tolerate our obsession with work. In short, we Americans deserve to live better, and we need to for the sake of our health, our happiness, and all those around us.

KNOW YOUR LIFESTYLE STATS

If you came to the Pritikin Center, one of the first things you would be asked to do is outline (or, in some cases, admit) your current lifestyle and health status. Shortly after your arrival, we would do a complete physical exam and lab analysis. This is where we start, because those are the true indexes of health. As the old saying goes, you don't know where you need to go until you know where you are to begin with. We have a team of some of the finest doctors, exercise physiologists, nutritionists, and psychologists in the world that would assess your health from every angle.

Since you're likely reading this book from the comfort of your living room rather than the Pritikin campus, we'll have to quiz you on your lifestyle stats on paper instead. You're on the honor system, now—no cheating!

Ask yourself these questions:

1. Do you weigh more than 155 pounds at five feet six inches tall, more than 169 pounds at five foot nine, or more than 184 pounds at six feet? If so, you are overweight. Sorry, but it's true. Obesity is a fast track to heart disease, diabetes, and depression.
2. Is your weight concentrated around your middle? Pick up a tape measure. A waist greater than 40 inches in a man or 35 inches in a woman is the unhealthiest form of obesity.
3. Are Big Macs, fries, and shakes a staple of your diet? Do they

know you by name at the local KFC? Just walking into a fast-food joint at least twice a week doubles your chance of getting diabetes.

4. On the subject of slow suicide, do you smoke? For every minute that you smoke, you shorten your life by one minute. (And while we're at it, if your answer to this question was yes, where have you been the last 40 years?!?)

5. Is your cholesterol greater than 150? That may sound like a low number, but anything over 150 can cause heart disease.

6. Is your blood pressure 120/80 or higher? If so, you officially have high blood pressure, which leads to stroke, kidney disease, and heart disease.

7. Are you physically inactive? (Hint: if there's an indentation on your couch from your backside, chances are you're not getting enough exercise!)

8. Are you and those around you pessimistic, stressed, or angry much of the time? Emotional problems very often become physical problems, including heart disease.

If you cannot say a hearty no to all these questions, a lifestyle overhaul is in order. You're not alone, though; fewer than 10 percent of Americans score perfectly on this test. The good news is that there's plenty of room for improvement!

CASE STUDY: MARGARET'S FIRST VISIT

Throughout this book, you are going to meet real patients who have changed their lives for the better. Except for well-known individuals, I have left off their surnames to protect their privacy. Here you'll meet Margaret, whom you'll get to know pretty well. I'll tell you about her first visit now, and about her three subsequent visits later. Her story illustrates how one motivated individual translated the Pritikin philosophy and practices into a better lifestyle.

Margaret came to see me concerned about her weight and the possibility of heart disease. With curly brown hair and an open, friendly smile, Margaret looked a lot like many people all of us know and love. As the married mother of two with a full-time job as a paralegal, Margaret's life was busy, and she often ate on the run (sound familiar?). Though she was not chubby as a child and weighed 132 pounds when she got married, Margaret gained 10 pounds with each of her children, and the rest accumulated slowly over the next 20 years. She had already tried several popular diets, but failed to keep off any of the weight she lost. Her mother had died of a heart attack at 58, an age that Margaret was rapidly approaching. Her grandfather had died suddenly even younger.

Fortunately, Margaret did not have any symptoms pointing to heart disease. I didn't find anything overly worrisome when I examined her, except that she stood 5 feet 4 inches tall and weighed 172 pounds—an all too typical American combination. Margaret carried most of her extra 40 pounds around her waist, which measured a not-so-svelte 37 inches. Her blood pressure was 138 over 86, which she had been told was normal (it isn't; it's too high). I ordered a cholesterol panel and a fasting blood sugar, but I already knew that Margaret needed to lose weight and lower her blood pressure if she wanted to get on a heart-healthy track.

On her first visit, I went through my Pritikin checklist of reasons why people are overweight:

1. I asked Margaret how often she drank high-calorie beverages, such as regular soda, fruit juice, coffee with sugar and cream, and alcohol. Happily, this wasn't an issue. She drank only water or diet soda and used low-calorie sweetener in her coffee. At most, she drank two glasses of wine on Fridays and Saturdays when she dined out with her husband. I marked "OK" next to beverages.

2. I asked some specifics about her diet, most specifically about two of the cornerstones of the Pritikin diet: salads and soups. Margaret told me that she had a salad two or three times a week for lunch and always a small salad and vegetables with dinner. But, like many people, she was drowning her salad in high-fat dressing (two packets equals a whopping 400 calories) and sprinkled cheese (another 100 calories). In reality, her salads were the dietary equivalent of cheeseburg-

ers camouflaged by a few greens. As for soups, Margaret liked the canned variety, such as chicken and minestrone. In the cattle world, these would be considered salt licks. I wrote "needs a little help with salad dressing and salt."

3. Next, we talked about calorie-dense foods—that is, foods packed with calories. Margaret asked what that meant. The exact definition of calorie-dense is having more than 500 calories per pound of food. It's a safe bet that any foods preferred by teenagers or sold in fast-food franchises are calorie-dense. Meats, cheese, chips, junk food, and desserts are calorie-dense. By contrast, fruits, vegetables, and soups are generally calorie-light. I tried to get a sense of her portions of calorie-dense foods. Did she eat half a bagel scraped with margarine for breakfast, or a whole bagel laden with cream cheese? (Answer: the whole bagel.) Did she regularly eat at fast-food restaurants? (Answer: at least twice a week.) Did she polish off her steak, French fries, and death-by-chocolate dessert when she ate out, or would she routinely leave food on her plate and/or take home a doggy bag? Like many of us, Margaret's mother must have taught her to clean her plate, because she never left anything, even in restaurants notorious for humongous entrée and dessert portions. (Rule of thumb: if a plate is bigger than your torso, It's too much food.) I noted "needs help with caloric density."

4. What about snacking? Did Margaret keep junk food around the house and office? Did she snack while driving or watching TV? Was a movie not quite the same experience for her without Milk Duds and a tub of buttered popcorn? I often don't get an honest answer to that question, but Margaret maintained that she didn't have a sweet tooth and that she rarely snacked at work or home. She got an "OK" on snacks.

5. Lastly, we discussed exercise. Margaret had played high school tennis and did aerobics when she was first married, but like so many busy people, stopped all exercise after she had her first child. She drove to and from work and sat long hours at her desk. Instead of walking her dog like she used to, she simply let her out into the backyard in the morning. Evenings were spent in front of the TV, or curled

up with a good mystery novel. I wrote and underlined <u>"couch potato"</u> next to exercise.

Like many of the people we see at Pritikin, Margaret thought that she ate reasonable amounts of pretty good food. She didn't understand why she continued to gain weight, especially because she liked salads, drank only diet beverages, and never snacked. Still, Margaret was not following three key weight-loss essentials that we teach: limiting calorie-dense foods, avoiding fast food, and getting daily exercise. She also needed to eat more and better salads and soups and cut down on her salt intake. Although she was practicing some of the Pritikin essentials (she didn't smoke, and seemed to manage her stress level well), I explained that she needed to start practicing *all* of them if she wanted to get her health on track.

We went to work. I told Margaret that, assuming she was typical of our Pritikin guests, she could expect to shed about ten pounds in the first three weeks if she followed my recommendations. After that, I didn't want her to lose any more than three to four pounds each month until she reached her goal of 40 pounds. It would probably take her about a year to do this, which was fine with me; the goal here was not just to lose the weight, but to *keep it off for good*.

We started by tackling the calorie-density issue. I outlined a diet of calorie-light salads, soups, whole grains, vegetables, and fruit, and instructed her to cut back on calorie-dense, refined carbs and fatty foods. I assured her she would not be hungry.

"How many calories a day should I eat?" Margaret wanted to know.

My answer surprised her. I told her I didn't want her to count calories.

"Then how will I know if I'm eating too much?" she protested.

"Simple," I said. "You won't be losing weight."

My instructions for Margaret included filling up with bigger salads for lunch and dinner. Emphasis on BIGGER! (I joked that the salad bowls at the Pritikin Center come with diving boards at one end.) She could add beans and other vegetables to the salad, but needed to leave off the cheese and fat-laden dressing, or better yet, convert to low-calorie dressings, lemon juice, or tasty balsamic vinegar. If she started with a big salad, she would naturally eat less calorie-dense food later in the meal, and thus lose weight. The science is simple: 100 fewer calories per day means 10 pounds lighter in a year.

I told her to forget fast food of any kind. If she was in a hurry, she should go to the deli section of a supermarket, where she could better control her food portions and ingredients. My friend Dr. Bill Castelli quips that when you go through the "golden arches," the "pearly gates" aren't far behind. That resonated with Margaret, especially in view of her mother's history.

As for salt, I told Margaret to season her food with anything but. Other spices, lemon juice, and vinegar were fine.

Lastly, I told her to invest $20 in a pedometer and measure how much she walked each day for a week. Then she needed to increase her total walking by 3,500 steps, or about two miles a day. Again, simple math: one more mile walked per day means 10 pounds lighter in a year.

The whole visit took less than an hour. Margaret took her instructions and headed out the door, filled with determination. I told her to come back and see me in a month to see how she was doing.

Stay tuned.

Your Lifestyle IQ

As you can see from Margaret's story, often we think we know more about what's healthy than we really do. Let's test your lifestyle knowledge.

1. Which is healthier for you, olive oil or canola oil?
2. What is the best dietary advice for your heart: eat less fat, eat more fiber, or eat more fish?
3. How much more would you weigh in five years if you ate one more 100-calorie cookie every day?
4. Which contains more sodium, a portion of cornflakes or a portion of potato chips?
5. Who describes his or her life as less enjoyable, an obese child or a child with cancer?

6. Who benefits more from exercise, a middle-aged person or an elderly person?
7. Is happiness life-saving?

Question 1: *Which is healthier for you, olive oil or canola oil?*

Everyone knows that olive oil is good for your heart. Right? Surprisingly, it's actually the omega-3 loaded oils, such as canola, walnut, flaxseed, and fish oils, that have been proven in scientific studies to save lives. Olive oil is better than butter, for sure, but canola oil is even better.

Question 2: *What is the best dietary advice for your heart: eat less fat, eat more fiber, or eat more fish?*

In a large British trial, eating less fat, more fiber, and more fish were compared. Eating less fat and more fiber had no effect on mortality, but eating more fish reduced deaths by about 30 percent, mostly because it reduced heart disease. Eating more fish and other omega-3 rich foods is the best dietary advice for your heart.

Question 3: *How much more would you weigh in five years if you ate one more 100-calorie cookie every day?*

What's a measly little 100 calories, right? Well, consider this: one additional 100-calorie cookie per day is almost one added pound per month. In five years, you would add 50 pounds just by eating an extra cookie every day.

Ultimately, that is terrific news, because it tells you how easy it is to lose weight, even if slowly. Take just one cookie out of your diet and you will lose 50 pounds in five years. We recognize, of course, that you neither want to get thin nor rich slowly. You want to be rich and thin by next Thursday. The truth is that you have almost as much chance of winning a lottery as permanently losing weight by crash dieting.

Question 4: *Which contains more sodium, a portion of cornflakes or a portion of potato chips?*

One ounce of cornflakes contains more than 200 milligrams of sodium, even before you add milk. Potato chips vary by manufacturer, but generally contain between 120 and 180 milligrams of sodium per ounce. Most of the high blood pressure generating sodium in our diet is hidden in processed foods we never think of as salty. Canned food and soups are especially loaded with sodium.

Question 5: *Who describes his or her life as less enjoyable, an obese child or a child with cancer?*

Obesity in America has exploded in the last 20 to 30 years. Teenagers today are 31 pounds heavier than they were 30 years ago. This is a huge medical problem because, as we already know, obesity is the fastest path to heart disease, high blood pressure, stroke, and diabetes.

Jolly fat people exist only in fairy tales. In a recent study, obese children ranked their quality of life on par with children undergoing treatment for cancer. Obesity is anything but enjoyable.

Question 6: *Who benefits more from exercise, a middle-aged person or an elderly person?*

The FDA would approve the drug equivalent of exercise in about two minutes flat. Physical activity not only reduces obesity, it slows aging and picks up our spirits. We live an hour longer for every hour we spend physically active.

Unfortunately, we have become the ultimate sedentary society. We endlessly circle parking lots looking for the closest parking spot. We panic when we lose the remote control and—heaven forbid!—actually have to stand up to change the channel. Our children play video games rather than outdoor games.

Yes, our children need to be more physically active, but the original question was about us old farts out there, who are the ones who benefit the most from exercise. In the Honolulu Heart study, middle-aged men had 17 percent less heart disease if they walked 30 minutes daily, but elderly men had 50 percent less heart disease. The older we get, the more we need to exercise.

Question 7: *Is happiness life-saving?*

You already know that stress is unhealthy. Sudden deaths triple in the year after a spouse's demise; Mondays and earthquakes both double the incidence of heart attacks. Just as stress, anger, and social isolation accelerate heart disease, joy and mirth can impede its attack. The bottom line here is that the head is connected to the heart in more ways than one. Enjoying life is a great way to keep your ticker strong and healthy.

Happy Life, Healthy Heart

- In one 10-year study, 1,300 men were evaluated on their optimism. The most optimistic men turned out to have half as many heart problems as the pessimistic men.
- In a recent Dutch study of elderly individuals, the happiest participants were half as likely to die over a nine-year period. In other words, the pessimists were twice as likely to kick the bucket.
- In a four-year study, 189 heart-failure patients who were happily married died half as frequently as those in unhappy marriages.

How did you do on these questions? If you answered all seven correctly, congratulations! If you got some of them wrong, it's perfectly understandable; most of us don't have the facts in hand that can improve and lengthen our lives. The good news is that they are all here in these pages.

START TODAY, IMPROVE TOMORROW

Some of my patients look at me when I talk about lifestyle as if to ask, "How much time do I have before I really need to start listening to you?" I remind them that a weekend of salads does not immediately undo years of cheese-steak hoagies. Meaningful, long-term changes make big differences, however. If you quit smoking at age 30, the probability is that you will live three to five years longer. When I tell that to my 30-year-old smokers, they tell me that they are not interested in living to 80. Who would want to live to 80? For starters, my 79-year-old patients certainly do.

The most compelling reason for starting heart-healthy lifestyle practices at a younger age is that you probably have not yet had a heart attack or stroke. Two-thirds of the time, the first symptom of heart disease is a heart attack—or worse. Even if you survive your first bout with heart disease, you will be six times more likely to have a rematch.

If you already have heart disease, fortunately, the better lifestyle choices you make as of this moment will significantly lower your risk of having another life-threatening event. Just as with obesity, preventing heart disease is much easier than treating it.

Trust me, I'm not telling you all this from some doctoral ivory tower. I've lived with the loss of loved ones who didn't take care of themselves. My father-in-law never experienced chest pains; sudden cardiac death was the first sign that he really should quit smoking and bring down his blood pressure. He was 59 years old. So far he has missed the whole of his retirement, three grandchildren, and three great-grandchildren. And those great-grandkids are really cute. If you don't believe me, I'll gladly send pictures.

CASE STUDY: DANNY, 89 YEARS OLD/YOUNG

Danny was a young track athlete at Michigan State in the 1940s. He has raced with the best of the best, even having had the honor of losing to Jesse Owens.

By the early 1980s, as a top insurance agent, Danny was doing a different kind of running, working 10- to 14-hour days, eating on the run or not at all, and giving up his jogging schedule to make it all fit in. In 1982, the 64-year-old dynamo suffered a heart attack. Bypass surgery was suggested.

Danny refused the surgery, but life was lousy. He was depressed, scared, and bored. Concerned, his rabbi handed him an article about the Pritikin Longevity Center. In April 1983, Danny arrived at Pritikin. The first few days, he couldn't walk more than a block. But at the end of his 26-day program, he was logging 12 to 14 miles daily. His stress tests improved, his cholesterol plummeted from 285 to 147, and his weight dropped from 176 pounds to 159, just three pounds over his college weight.

It's now 25 years since that first visit to Pritikin. Danny returns regularly to the center. He takes no medications and has never had another heart problem. Four days a week, he runs three miles. Twice weekly, he lifts weights with a personal trainer. And three days a week, he still takes care of clients, supervising one office in Florida and another in Connecticut.

"In those three days, I accomplish more than I used to accomplish in seven," laughs the spry 89-year-old. "I'm still a young man!"

KEY POINTS TO REMEMBER

- Heart disease is best prevented through lifestyle changes.
- For optimal results, you need to adopt *all* of the 10 Pritikin lifestyle essentials.
- Lifestyle changes are far preferable to medications.
- You need to know your lifestyle stats to enable you to understand and appreciate fully *why* you are making these essential lifestyle changes.
- Get started today. The sooner you start living better, the more significantly you reduce your risk of having a life-threatening coronary event—and the greater your chances are of living that long, delicious life that made you pick up this book in the first place!

2

The Heart of the Matter

PLEASE DO NOT skip this chapter because it sounds complicated. We promise you, we've taken the confusion out of heart disease for many, many patients and participants in the Pritikin Program. What we teach them—and what we'll give you in this chapter—is the real science of heart disease that goes beyond the simplistic (and often untrue) descriptions found in most popular lifestyle books. Here, and throughout the book, you'll come to understand the *why* behind our lifestyle advice; this is valuable because the more you know and understand about heart disease and its risk factors, the more motivated you'll be to make those lifestyle changes we've been talking about, once and for all.

First, let's start with the language of heart disease. *Cardiovascular disease* is the umbrella term for heart disease, stroke, and high blood pressure. All the other terms may sound complex and scary, but once you know what they are, you'll see they are just the mechanical words we use to describe various parts and functions in your body. For the purposes of this book, there are basically 12 terms you need to know in order to feel (and sound) educated when it comes to matters of the heart.

Dictionary of Cardiovascular Disease

Angina pectoris: the medical term for chest pain.

Atherosclerosis: a common disease that progressively blocks arteries; commonly referred to as "hardening of the arteries."

Cholesterol: a complex molecule that is an important ingredient of cell walls and hormones (broken down into two types: LDL, or "bad" cholesterol, which gets deposited in your arteries, and HDL, or "good" cholesterol, which is being returned to your liver to be excreted).

Coronary arteries: the three major blood vessels and their branches that supply blood to the heart muscle so it can work as a pump.

Coronary risk factors: characteristics that contribute to the likelihood of developing atherosclerosis, including high cholesterol and high blood pressure.

Endothelium: the single-cell-thick inner lining of your blood vessels.

Inflammation: the process by which tissues respond to injuries such as trauma or infection.

Myocardial infarction: also known as a heart attack or coronary occlusion; it is the death of heart muscle that usually results from a sudden decrease in blood flow through a coronary artery.

Nitric oxide: a simple molecule made by the endothelium that expands blood vessels and retards the development of atherosclerosis. Considered a protective chemical in the body.

Plaque: a local buildup of atherosclerosis in the artery wall.

Stroke: the death of brain tissue that usually results from a sudden decrease in blood flow to the brain.

Thrombosis: also known as a blood clot; the immediate cause of a heart attack or stroke.

UNDERSTANDING ATHEROSCLEROSIS

Atherosclerosis, or hardening of the arteries, is the most common car-diovascular disease. About 80 percent of the heart disease that I see and treat in my cardiology practice falls into this classification. The word *atherosclerosis* comes from a combination of the Greek *athero*, for gruel or porridge, and *sclerosis*, for hardening. Thus, "hardening of the arter-ies" is an apt description.

Atherosclerosis was a relatively uncommon disease until the Indus-trial Revolution, which decreased the need for physical work and made food abundant. Until about 100 years ago, people were paid to do hard physical work and food was relatively expensive. Now, food is cheap and you have to pay for sneakers and health clubs to get some exercise. We remain genetically encoded to be active hunter-gatherers; unfortunately, we now hunt in fast-food restaurants and gather in malls. Will natural selection eventually make people more atherosclerosis resistant? Proba-bly not. Most heart disease occurs after the child-bearing years, giving little gene selection advantage to those who don't get heart disease. After we have children, the survival of our species depends on a healthy life-style, not Darwin.

Atherosclerosis can start at a very young age but may not produce symptoms for decades. Newborn babies of mothers with high choles-terol already have atherosclerosis. It's been shown that up to 60 percent of 25-year-old Americans killed in motor vehicle accidents or wars al-ready have some evidence of atherosclerosis in their arteries. Five to 10 percent of young adults in this country already have a substantial plaque in at least one coronary artery. The youngest patient I have sent to bypass surgery because of lifestyle-induced coronary artery narrowing was 22 years old at the time. Atherosclerosis starts much earlier than you think.

How Do Our Arteries "Harden"?

Here's how atherosclerosis happens, in a nutshell (and here's where your glossary of heart disease terms will come in handy). First, it's important to understand that the hardening, or narrowing, that occurs is a result of chronic injury to the arteries. We injure them through long-term wear and tear, such as high cholesterol and high blood pressure, what we call *coronary risk factors.*

High cholesterol injures the arteries by affecting the biology of the walls of the blood vessels in two important ways: it reduces the protective chemicals, including *nitric oxide,* and increases *inflammatory* ones (nitric oxide = good; inflammation = bad). Inflammation, which we'll explain in more detail a little later in this chapter, basically is a process by which the body responds to injury; when you cut your skin and the area gets warm and swollen, that is the result of white blood cells rushing to the area to promote healing. However, sustained or excessive inflammation creates a scarring effect in the arteries by thickening the tissue. Obesity, which we'll talk about more in the next chapter, further contributes to inflammation, because the stuffed fat cells in your belly actually make and release the inflammatory chemicals.

Additionally, the bad (LDL) cholesterol gets deposited in the arteries, and that sets off a reaction. Like an oyster responding to a grain of sand within, the body reacts. Instead of getting a pearl, though, we get a slew of white blood cells rushing to the site to eat the cholesterol. Just like Great Uncle Murray at Thanksgiving, they can and will stuff themselves; unlike Great Uncle Murray, though (at least I hope), these engorged cells can burst and do a lot of damage.

High blood pressure, too, injures the arteries, through the pounding of the pressure on the walls of your blood cells. All this leads to scarring along the walls of your arteries and local buildups known as *plaque.*

So, what's the tipping point? One day, a plaque will ulcerate (i.e. rupture) and form a clot, also called a *thrombus*, inside your arteries. When clots form, one of two things will happen: if your arteries have narrowed substantially but aren't totally blocked, you'll experience chest pain. If the blockage is total, however, you'll have a heart attack or, if the clot and blockage is in an artery leading to your brain, a stroke.

Over decades, atherosclerosis builds up inside arteries at a varying pace. There may be no change in the narrowing for years, and then, at other times, it may progress very rapidly and occur at multiple sites. Narrowing at any site in the body (say, the carotid artery in the neck or the aorta, the large artery coming out of the heart) makes it much more likely that it will happen at other sites. Thus, having a stroke means you are more likely to have a heart attack at some point, and vice versa.

The chronic nature of atherosclerosis is fortuitous because it gives us time to slow down the narrowing process. Once the pace of atherosclerosis stops, heart attacks and strokes become much less likely, even if the narrowing remains. We are even learning how to reverse the plaque buildup through intensive lifestyle and drug treatments.

The Myth of "Clogged" Arteries

Atherosclerosis is *not* similar to the corrosion inside water pipes. That is a much-quoted though highly inaccurate analogy. In truth, atherosclerosis involves cholesterol deposits along the artery walls, but most of the narrowing is caused by a buildup of fibrous (scar) tissue that formed in response to repeated trauma.

Am I implying that atherosclerosis is the body's natural response to injury? Yes! The "response-to-injury" hypothesis has been our basic understanding of this disease for almost 150 years. We are not clogging our arteries, but injuring them. Atherosclerosis is an active process, not a passive one.

The Role of Nitric Oxide

Nitric oxide is a very simple but important molecule. It is not the same as *nitrous oxide,* or "laughing gas." The nitric oxide story is no laughing matter; it will determine how long you live.

Nitric oxide is made by the blood vessels' lining, or *endothelium.* The endothelium is exquisitely sensitive to the physical and chemical conditions inside our blood vessels. When the endothelium senses heart-healthy conditions, such as physical activity and low cholesterol, it releases more nitric oxide. Nitric oxide expands the blood vessels, increasing blood flow and decreasing plaque growth and blood clotting. Conversely, when the endothelium senses high cholesterol, high blood pressure, smoking, or emotional distress, it releases less nitric oxide, and atherosclerosis accelerates.

Attention, Gentlemen!

Penile erection depends on the release of nitric oxide. Viagra and other drugs like it that reduce erectile dysfunction work on the next step of the nitric oxide pathway. Are impotence and atherosclerosis closely related? Absolutely. Any lifestyle no-no that decreases nitric oxide, such as smoking, causes both problems.

Nitroglycerin, which my grandfather took to relieve his chest pain, works by being converted into nitric oxide. In a sense, nitric oxide is the body's own nitroglycerin. If you had first discovered how nitroglycerin and nitric oxide work, as three Americans (Robert Furchgott, Lewis Ignarro, and Ferid Murad) did, in 1998 you would have won the Nobel Prize for Medicine. Nitric oxide is that important.

Inflammation

In many situations, inflammation is helpful, if not life-saving: when we are injured, for instance, or when we have a virus or other infection. The body naturally responds, as you already know, by rushing white blood cells to the area to begin damage control. Scar tissue is accelerated, which heals cuts and scrapes. Without inflammation, we could neither survive the simplest sinus infection nor close the smallest paper cut. In our evolutionary history, a vigorous inflammation response gave us a survival advantage, because infections and injury were more of a threat. Today, with antibiotics readily abundant and fewer wild tigers on the loose, unchecked inflammation is left to cause many degenerative diseases including atherosclerosis, Alzheimer's, and arthritis.

The only difference between inflammation of the regular sort and the kind that triggers atherosclerosis is that high cholesterol, high blood pressure, smoking, and obesity are initiating the inflammation, not infection or trauma. Unlike a brief infection or trauma, these risk factors are longstanding and therefore lead to chronic inflammation and plaque. Active plaques begin to resemble small abscesses on the inside of arteries. These active plaques are thought to be sites of future heart attacks.

Your Arteries Know How You Live!

Now that you know more about the real science of heart disease, consider just a few factors about the link between the lifestyle changes we recommend and your heart health:

- We strongly recommend canola oil over the current popular favorite, olive oil, for dressing your salads and cooking. Why? Because olive oil actually lowers your body's release of nitric oxide and canola oil doesn't. Moreover, canola oil reduces inflammation much more than olive oil. Yes, really!
- Exercise not only gives your heart a workout and burns off yesterday's pasta; it also pumps your nitric oxide and reduces inflammation.
- Watching a scary movie reduces nitric oxide in your arteries, but funny movies increase it. Like Santa Claus, your arteries know whether you've been naughty or nice.

Coronary Risk Factors

We have known for more than 50 years that certain characteristics make atherosclerosis more likely. The major risk factors are:

- Older age (45 years for men and 55 years for women)
- Male sex
- High cholesterol
- High blood pressure
- Smoking
- Diabetes
- Family history of early heart disease

Much of our information on risk factors comes from the Framingham Heart Study, which was initiated in 1948. Observation is the first step in medical science, so in that and other similar studies, healthy individuals were observed over many years to determine which factors led to heart disease. From these studies, we have learned that these seven risk factors are directly responsible for about 90 percent of heart disease.

In two recent reviews of more than 150,000 people with heart disease, a whopping 85 percent had high cholesterol, high blood pressure, diabetes, and/or were smokers. The good news is that these are four critical risk factors we can change. We can't do much about being born of the male persuasion, or our family history, but reducing our cholesterol, blood pressure, and diabetes risk and quitting smoking are absolutely within our control. Dozens of studies have found that treating these risk factors lessens heart disease. And, most important, many trials have proven that lifestyle changes are among the most effective treatments. Unlike cancer, we know exactly what causes heart disease and how to prevent it. We've been doing it successfully at the Pritikin Longevity Center for 30 years.

The Number-One Risk Factor You Can Change

Among the risk factors for heart disease, high cholesterol takes the prize as the single most important modifiable factor. Why? Because excess blood cholesterol first seeps into the arterial wall. Free cholesterol does not belong there, and the body reacts to it the same way that it reacts to splinters. In response to the "injury," white blood cells migrate to the area, where they eat the cholesterol deposits. Some actually eat so much that they die and burst, causing more damage. The released cholesterol forms small abscesses, similar to the way an abscess forms around a splinter in your skin. Cholesterol lying around in the walls of arteries ages, like food left in the back of the refrigerator. Aged cholesterol is better recognized by white blood cells as a foreign invader, and the process of inflammation is perpetuated.

Chest Pain

We are lucky that atherosclerosis usually builds up slowly. The slow development allows the diseased arteries to enlarge, as if to preserve the remaining open channel. This compensation keeps blood flowing almost normally during the first decades of atherosclerosis. Unfortunately, though, it cannot keep up forever. When the open channel becomes severely narrowed, blood flow to the heart muscle is impeded—especially during exercise, when more blood is needed. The result is chest pain, medically termed *angina pectoris*.

Chest pain during exercise is a troubling symptom; it is a warning that heart attack may be in your near future. To be frank, so might sudden death if you don't pay attention. Chest pain means you need to seek immediate medical care—and that you need to start changing how you live *today*. Consider chest pain your body's final warning that you're at serious risk.

What to Do if You Experience Chest Pain

1. Put down the cheeseburger.
2. Call 911 immediately.
3. Read and start living the 10 essential ingredients in Part Two of this book—*as soon as possible.* You're being given a second chance at living a long, healthy life.

KEY POINTS TO REMEMBER

- Heart attacks and strokes are caused by a blockage in the arteries that prevents blood flow to the heart or brain.
- We do not clog our arteries; we essentially narrow them through chronic injury that creates scar tissue.
- High blood pressure, high cholesterol, smoking, and obesity cause the chronic arterial injury by decreasing nitric oxide release and increasing inflammation.
- Reducing your cholesterol is the single best thing you can do to retard the process of atherosclerosis.
- Chest pain is a serious warning that you need to seek medical treatment and make some lifestyle changes immediately.

3

The Weight/Health Connection

WE AMERICANS ARE now the fattest people on Earth. Yes, that's right: *on the planet*. The occasional sumo wrestler in Japan aside, we hold the record for global obesity. Sixty-six percent of us are overweight, and 32 percent of us are truly obese. On average, we weigh 20 percent more than we should. And we certainly eat more than we should. Some of us eat too much refined carbohydrates, such as sugar and white bread. Some of us eat too much fat. Some eat too much junk and fast food. Most of us just eat too much of everything.

The stats on obesity in this country are alarming. Severe obesity has quadrupled over the past 20 years. The 1990s were especially fat years for America: between 1991 and 1998, obesity increased 50 percent in adults and 70 percent in children. All measures of weight gain continue to expand even now. Two percent more Americans achieved overweight status in the time it took us to write this book.

Is it our genes, our metabolism, or our lifestyle? The very recent increase in obesity gives us important clues. Since our genes and metabolism could not have evolved that much in the past few years, they clearly can't be the culprit. We're fatter now primarily because of our lifestyle, plain and simple.

One of the questions patients ask almost without fail is, "But aren't some people more prone to becoming obese?" They point to their Great Aunt Harriet, who topped the scale at 300, or their entire family tree, whose branches are drooping with plus-sized relatives. Our answer to them is that certainly, some people are more prone to being overweight. But there's more to the story than just that. Keep reading!

During human evolution, storing calories as fat gave us a survival advantage because food was not always available. The set of genes that drive us to eat more when food is available and to store food efficiently are called "thrifty genes." Seventy percent of African-Americans, 50 percent of Asians, and 30 percent of Caucasians have these thrifty genes. These very genes that millions of years ago were our ticket to survival are now killing us, because we don't *need* to store food. The nearest supermarket or stocked refrigerator is, for most of us, not more than a few steps away. Even so, possessing these "thrifty genes" does not guarantee obesity; having them just means we need to exercise more lifestyle discipline to remain slim.

Why Are We So Fat?

The period from the late 1970s to the late 1990s was a boon for the food industry. During these years, we Americans increased our daily food consumption by 194 calories, of which 148 came from snacks. One hundred and ninety-four calories doesn't sound like a lot, but it is largely responsible for our epidemic of obesity. What in our culture made us eat more and gain more so fast? We've boiled it down to six factors:

- Food costs less because of more efficient production and longer shelf life.

- Food is more widely available and there are more food varieties from which to choose.
- Food portions have grown considerably larger.
- We eat prepared and restaurant meals more because in more households, both adults/parents work.
- We drink far more sugar-laden beverages.
- Fewer of us lead active lifestyles, and fewer jobs require physical activity.

Pretend that you are in the food industry. Your job is to sell food. What would you do? You would try to make food cheaper and more widely available, create a lot of varieties, and make it tasty. That is exactly what the food industry has done. Industrial farming is much more efficient at producing food cheaply than family farming. It's a simple question of scale. Many foods are still prepared with trans fats, which keep them fresh longer on the shelf. Trans fats are real killers; gram for gram, they have even more impact on our heart health than offending saturated fats. Why? Because they managed to not only raise our bad cholesterol, but also reduce our good cholesterol. Foods containing trans fats may stay fresh longer, but you won't. Better packaging also extends freshness, and the longer foods last, the lower their cost. The lower the cost, the more we eat.

Food is not only cheap nowadays; it is available everywhere in great variety. In marketing-speak, these principles are called exposure and choice. With so many options and tastes out there, we're driven to sample and consume more. Snack and junk food varieties have increased the most, and are responsible for about three-quarters of our increased caloric intake.

Food portion sizes have grown to obscene proportions. The six-ounce cola bottle of my childhood is now a collector's item. The food industry has learned that people will eat more simply if more food is put in front of them. This is the "super-sizing" principle popularized by fast-food chains. Eating more is wonderful for growth within the food industry, not so wonderful for the expansion of our waistlines. Eating more makes us fat, period. We then need to eat even more to maintain our fatter bodies.

The food industry has also discovered that inexpensive high-fructose corn syrup tastes 30 percent sweeter than regular sugar. Since we innately love sweet food (yours truly is as guilty as anyone!), we will eat and drink more foods with added high-fructose corn syrup. The problem is that high-fructose corn syrup doesn't turn off our hunger mechanism very efficiently, so we just keep eating. And eating, and eating.

None of this is a food industry conspiracy. Remember, their job is to sell more food. Our job is to teach you how to eat fewer calories without having to go hungry or sacrificing satiety. Let's start with some motivation.

THE CONSEQUENCES OF OBESITY

If you're reading this book, there's a good chance that I'm not the first doctor to warn you about the health consequences of being overweight. If you're reading it preventatively, congratulations—that's wonderful! Either way, we at Pritikin believe it's vitally important for patients to understand exactly why they need to lose weight in order for them to stay motivated from within.

Let's start with the obvious: obesity is unattractive, socially isolating, and depressing. It markedly decreases quality of life. In one study, 27 percent of the unhappiness experienced by overweight individuals was traced to their obesity. Like it or not, obese individuals are thought of as lazy or lacking self-control. Standards of attractiveness vary, but obesity is generally considered a real turn-off. As our society gets fatter, we still continue to deride those among us who are obese. All dieters know how much better they feel after losing weight, and how demoralized they feel when they gain it back. Now multiply that by many more pounds, and you can understand why depression and low self-esteem are rampant among the obese.

Obesity also takes a toll on your health, especially your heart health.

Obesity causes cardiovascular disease in a number of ways. It increases blood pressure, LDL (bad) cholesterol, triglycerides, and blood sugar, and decreases HDL (good) cholesterol. Obesity reduces the liver's ability to clear cholesterol from the bloodstream and impairs the sugar-lowering response to insulin. Overly stuffed fat deposits, especially inside the abdomen, release several hormones that increase inflammation and decrease nitric oxide.

Obesity also makes it more difficult to be physically active and, as we already know, gets in the way of our ability to feel emotionally upbeat. Remember, all these are risk factors that initiate—and then promote—atherosclerosis.

Obesity 101

Here are a few general facts about the risks of obesity worth knowing:

- Heart attacks increase about 2 percent for each 1 percent increase in LDL (bad) cholesterol. Obesity can increase bad cholesterol by as much as 50 percent.
- Heart disease increases about 2 percent for every 1 percent decrease in good cholesterol. Obesity lowers good cholesterol by 20 to 30 percent.
- Diabetic levels of blood sugar, which are usually caused by obesity, are associated with a threefold increase in heart disease.
- Obesity directly injures the endothelium, or lining of your blood vessels, and causes inflammation. As weight increases, so does inflammation. Fat, especially inside the abdomen, stokes the fires of inflammation, just like adding coal to a stove.
- Obese individuals who lose 30 pounds decrease markers of inflammation by about 50 percent.
- Nitric oxide levels fall off sharply in individuals weighing more than ap-

(continued)

proximately 165 pounds at five feet six inches tall and more than 195 pounds at six feet tall.

- The leading preventable cause of death, cigarette smoking, kills 435,000 Americans annually and costs $150 billion in health care. Obesity isn't far behind, killing almost as many Americans (400,000) and costing $117 billion in health care.
- The annual personal health-care costs for an obese individual are $700 higher than a non-obese person.
- For the first time, the average lifespan is decreasing in counties with especially high rates of obesity.

What Mice Know That We Don't

Are we really sure that obesity kills? Let's go through the scientific process. Observational studies indicate that obese people do have more heart disease, high blood pressure, diabetes, and cancer than thin people. Obesity definitely increases the bad cholesterol, blood pressure, and inflammation in our bodies and decreases the good cholesterol and nitric oxide. Still, are these clear and plausible explanations enough to recommend weight loss to an entire population? As a cardiologist, of course I'd say yes, but as an author, I want to bring the point home even more and give you the results of a tried-and-true randomized controlled trial.

Let's put some mice in a cage. Let's feed one group as much food as they want and restrict calories in the other group. (By the way, this experiment has been done many times with mice and other species, and the results have always been the same.) Which mice live longer?

Before you hear the answer, think for a moment about how you were brought up and/or how you may be bringing up your own children. How many times have you heard or said, "Finish your plate so you can grow up to be a big, strong . . ." or "There are people starving in . . ." or "If you finish your plate, you can have dessert." Does that sound familiar? It's been shown that only 15 percent of Americans do not encourage their children to overeat. The other 85 percent would be well served by knowing that the calorie-restricted animals in these key experiments always live longer. Mice live 20 percent longer if their calories are modestly restricted and 80 percent longer if they are severely restricted. I know this principle sounds backward, but we in the medical community are very sure of its truth.

"Terrific," you might be thinking. "But I'm not a mouse." Well, we can easily extrapolate these findings to people. A recent six-month study done by Louisiana State University tested the effects of mild, moderate, and severe calorie restriction along with exercise. The volunteers in the study behaved just like mice. The calorie-restricted groups experienced a decrease in metabolic rate, lower body temperature, greater sensitivity to insulin, and less DNA gene damage. In other words, every index pointed in the direction of a longer life.

What about overeating? If restricting calories increases longevity, does overeating have the reverse effect? The answer is yes. Another recent study, of nine-year-old girls, showed that obese girls were far more likely to start puberty at an early age than those who were of normal weight. Obese children appear to behave much like obese mice: their lives go by faster.

When we insist that our children finish all the food on their plates, we are really telling them, "Grow up to be big and strong at age 20, and have a coronary bypass operation at age 50." When a child doesn't finish his or her food, that child is probably just no longer hungry. You should give your child a hug and leave it at that. Telling children to disregard their biological checks and balances sends the message that they should eat everything in sight. Let's not lead our kids down the road to obesity, or teach them that our love and approval come with overeating.

Obesity in Children

Our youngsters are becoming obese at an alarming rate. Obesity-related (type 2) diabetes has increased 800 percent during the past decade in teenagers. I recently learned of a *two-year-old* with obesity-caused diabetes.

Overweight children and teenagers need to lose weight now, before their risk for high blood pressure and other heart disease risk factors take hold. Besides which, appearance is a major factor in young people's social lives and their self-esteem.

It's time to give our kids a fighting chance early in life, and change the American lifestyle to encourage childhood slimness. The drive-thru may be convenient, but at what physical and emotional cost to our kids?

AM I OBESE?

Obese isn't just another way of saying really fat. Well, okay, maybe it is, in our common lexicon, but medically, there are specific markers that enable us to know whether a person falls into the technical definition of *obese*.

There are two measures we use to determine where a person falls on the scale of normal to obese. The first is body-mass index, and the other is waist circumference (along with waist-to-hip ratio). Let me walk you through how to measure for both to see what your measurements reveal about you.

Body-Mass Index

The most common definition of obesity is based on a person whose body-mass index, or BMI, is 30 or greater. What does that mean, exactly? Let me explain.

Body-mass index is a measurement of weight relative to height. To calculate your BMI in pounds and inches, grab a calculator. First, multiply your weight in pounds by 703. Divide the result by your height in inches, and then divide this result again by your height in inches. The result is your BMI.

Let's take me, for instance. I weigh 140 pounds and stand five feet seven inches (or 67 inches) tall. So, here's my calculation:

1. 140 lbs. x 703 = 98,420
2. 98,420 ÷ 67" = 1469
3. 1469 ÷ 67" = 21.9
   The resulting number is 21.9, which is my BMI.

The medically "normal" BMI for most adult Americans is between 18.5 and 25. The Framingham (Massachusetts) Heart Study, begun in 1948, taught us that heart disease risk is lowest at a BMI of exactly 22.6 in men and 21.1 in women. This is the weight at which we are genetically programmed to be most healthy. Interestingly, it is very close to the weight of our ancestors, who worked harder physically and snacked less than we do. Above and below these values, several diseases increase and longevity shortens.

So, back to what your BMI says about you:

- You are considered "normal" weight if your BMI is between 18.5 and 24.9.
- You are overweight if your BMI is between 25 and 29.9.
- You are obese if your BMI is between 30 and 39.9.
- You are extremely obese if your BMI is 40 or more.

Gender does not matter in the definition of obesity, nor does body build. We are not a nation of large-framed people. We are simply fat, and working hard to deny our collective fatness. We have only to look at fashion for proof: a current size-six dress was called an eight or ten in the past. It's certainly exciting to suddenly fit into a smaller size, but somehow less so when you realize that it's actually *bigger* than your old size!

Measuring Your BMI

1. Multiply your weight in pounds by 703.
2. Divide the result by your height in inches.
3. Divide that result by your height in inches again. The resulting number is your BMI.

The Belly Barometer

Body-mass index is only a measure of weight relative to height. It doesn't take into account how much fat we have or its distribution. Both of these factors are important because it is really fat inside the abdomen that causes heart disease and diabetes. To put it another way, from a health perspective, fat in the gut is worse than fat in the butt. This potbelly fat (sometimes called central, truncal, or male-pattern obesity) is more metabolically active and is a major cause of chronic inflammation throughout the body. Some women I know rue their pear-shaped bodies, but from a medical standpoint, pear shapes are far better off than their apple-shaped counterparts.

The standard measurements of fat distribution are waist circumference and waist-to-hip ratio. To figure out yours, the only tool you'll need is a tape measure.

In reality, many people don't know where their waist is. Your belt size is not the same as your waist circumference. Men especially keep the same belt size even while adding a big potbelly. We physicians think of the waist as the precise anatomical point that comes into our offices first. Waist circumference is medically measured horizontally at your iliac crest (top of your hip bone) at the end of an exhalation (no sucking in your gut, please). However, the circumference around your belly button is a good approximation.

In America, more than 40 inches of waist circumference is considered too much for a man, and more than 35 inches too much for a woman. Height is not really a factor here. By the way, internationally, the markers of "too much" are 37 inches for a man and 32 inches for a woman; we're clearly more fat-tolerant than the rest of the world. Men of South Asian, Central American, Japanese, and Chinese heritage should have a waist circumference of less than 35 inches, because they typically develop a host of metabolic abnormalities with smaller waists than do men of African or European descent.

Acceptable Waist Measurements

- For a man: less than 40 inches around*
- For a woman: less than 35 inches around*

----

* For optimal health subtract 5 inches.

Waist-to-Hip Ratio

The waist-to-hip ratio is an even better index of future heart disease, because it takes into account your waist circumference in relation to your specific body frame. By determining the ratio of your belly to your hips (ideally, your belly is smaller), you'll know instantaneously whether you're carrying too much of a spare tire around your middle.

To calculate your waist-to-hip ratio, measure your waist circumference (again, the distance around where your belly button is) and then your hip circumference (the point where your hips have the widest dimension). Divide your waist measurement by your hip measurement and you get your ratio. For women, the ratio should be under .85; for men, it should be under 1. Anything over that and you're in the danger zone.

Measuring Your Waist-to-Hip Ratio

1. Measure your waist circumference.
2. Measure your hip circumference.
3. Divide your waist circumference by your hip circumference. The resulting number is your ratio.

THE BENEFITS OF LOSING WEIGHT

For all the doom and gloom we've imparted here about obesity and its life-threatening effects, we have one piece of fantastic news: there's an immediate way to reverse obesity. That's right . . . losing weight. Because obesity contributes so mightily to heart disease and other insidious diseases, this is a major cornerstone of what we teach at Pritikin. Thousands of people have come through the program over the past 30 years to learn the best and most effective ways to lose weight, improve their health, and increase their odds for a longer life, all of which you'll learn in this book. We base our knowledge, as I said, not on passing trends or fads but on more than 110 research studies demonstrating the numerous metabolic improvements from the Pritikin Diet & Exercise Program, so you know what you're getting is real and that the results will last.

By losing as little as 10 to 20 pounds, you can make a big difference in improving your blood pressure, cholesterol, and blood sugar levels (three of the risk factors that make up what we call "metabolic syndrome"). In a recent study, overweight individuals with mildly elevated blood-sugar levels developed full-blown diabetes 58 percent less frequently after they lost an average of just 15 pounds on a reduced-calorie, low-fat diet and exercised for half an hour at least five times each week, compared with those who did not lose weight or exercise. Another recently published study showed that just three weeks of diet and exercise therapy at the Pritikin Center reversed the clinical diagnosis of metabolic syndrome in half the men studied. These results were most impressive because the men didn't have to wait until they lost huge amounts of weight; after shedding just 6 to 10 pounds, they improved virtually *all* the factors that lead to heart disease and diabetes. Your body knows very rapidly that you're working toward a better lifestyle. Health measures, such as blood pressure and cholesterol, improve long before you need a smaller belt size.

Then, of course, there are the cosmetic and emotional reasons to lose weight. A lighter frame makes it far easier to be physically active, which of course is another huge health benefit and one of our 10 essentials. Plus, there's nothing that compares to the satisfaction of fitting into a pair of pants you haven't been able to button in years! Losing weight improves your self-image, sleeping habits, social interactions, and overall sense of well-being. We've watched the transformation happen thousands of times at Pritikin. In the next chapter, and throughout the book, you'll learn the specifics of how to lose weight so you, too, can look better, feel better . . . and most important, live better.

CASE STUDY: MICHAEL

Michael is an energetic 46-year-old businessman with the customary busy life that goes along with a successful career, marriage, and family. He lives in Pennsylvania, where he launched and now operates a security company. Michael loves nothing more than vacationing at the shore with his wife and two girls, now ages 9 and 13.

Fifteen years ago, Michael walked down the aisle at his wedding weighing 180 pounds, an acceptable weight for his six-foot frame. In just eight years, however, he ballooned to 265 pounds. It wasn't until his 60-year-old mother died suddenly of a heart attack that Michael woke up and realized that he was not invincible. "You suddenly realize how precious life is," Michael said, sitting in my office as I examined him. "I remember standing on my bathroom scale and saying, 'You dope, you would take a bullet for your kids, but you won't go on a diet for them? Something doesn't make sense here, and it's got to change *now*.'" I assured him that he was doing the best thing he could possibly do for himself and his family, which was to rein in his weight gain now before the negative effects accumulated.

Michael soon started the Pritikin Program, following all 10 of the essentials. Within one year, he lost 78 pounds and went from a size 44 waist to a 34. "I have this belt that I love, and I've had to put two extra holes in it to keep wearing it," he laughed. "That's a good problem to have!"

People always ask him, "Isn't it hard to give up the good life?" Michael tells them the new philosophy by which he lives: *that nothing tastes as good as being thin feels.*

"I really like what I see in the mirror," Michael said. "My eyes are clear, my skin coloring is great, and I've lost my second chin. What's most impressive is that I look as good on the inside as I do on the outside. My cholesterol, which at one point was 297, is now below 100.

"I really haven't given up the good life," he continued. "With the Pritikin Program, I can have just about everything I desire. It satisfies all my food cravings. For breakfast, I'll have a bowl of oatmeal with raisins and cinnamon, an egg-white omelet with veggie cheese and roasted vegetables, or a whole-wheat bagel. I can even combine small portions of all three, plus fruit. That's a big breakfast! For lunch and dinner, there are so many choices. I enjoy grilled seafood, baked potatoes, pastas, veggie burgers, big salads . . . all I have to do is stay away from the white starchy, sugary stuff, and that's not a problem. I don't walk around unsatisfied."

The best part of Michael's story is the impact his healthy lifestyle is having on his family. "I learned a lot of bad eating habits as a kid," he said. "It wasn't my parents' fault; it was simply their generation. Now my wife and I are raising our daughters in a totally different way. When we first became a Pritikin family, my younger daughter was only three, but she quickly jumped on the bandwagon, saying things like, 'Look, Daddy, I'm eating fruits and vegetables!' and 'Sugar is bad for you.' Both girls eat nonfat frozen yogurt instead of full-fat ice cream. The bottom line is that we want our kids to grow up learning the right habits so that they will never need to lose 80 pounds like I did."

KEY POINTS TO REMEMBER

- America is the fattest country on Earth.
- Obesity markedly decreases a person's quality of life and greatly increases his or her risk of heart disease and diabetes.
- Belly fat is more dangerous healthwise than lower body fat.
- Waist circumference and waist-to-hip ratio are the best way to determine obesity.
- By losing as little as 10 to 20 pounds, you can make a big difference in improving your blood pressure, cholesterol, and blood sugar levels—as well as your overall sense of emotional well-being.

4

The Science of Weight Loss

SALLIE IS A bright, beautiful, emotionally nourishing family physician. Two years ago, in her early 50s, she weighed 184 pounds and wore plus-size dresses. One day at a dance class, she looked in the mirror and saw her grandmother. Sallie decided right there on the spot to do something good for herself and commit to losing weight.

Sallie traded her customary bread and pasta diet for beans, fruits, vegetables, and nuts, all of which she loves. But she was also wise enough to know she needed to change her whole lifestyle, not just her diet. She became a dancing fool—hip-hop, dance recitals, the works. She started jogging and redid her backyard by hand, bush by bush, stone by stone. She installed a pull-up bar in a doorway and started doing one or two chin-ups every time she goes by. Now she walks several miles every day with her husband, who has also caught the weight-loss bug.

Today, Sallie is 134 pounds and wears a size 4. She is even more emotionally nourishing to those around her, and when she looks in the mirror, she likes what she sees. Her lifestyle overhaul had paid off.

Sallie was successful because she understood one of the most irre-futable scientific facts about weight loss: diets alone don't work. She knew better than to buy into any of the popular quick fixes like "give up carbs." If any simple diet change produced sustained weight loss, we as a culture would not be so obese, nor would we be spending $40 billion annually on weight loss.

There are many diets out there these days that promise easy solu-tions. But remember, weight gain/loss is a complex issue to which there are no one-size-fits-all, simple solutions. In a recent study published in the *Journal of the American Medical Association*, obese volunteers interested in losing weight randomly went on one of the following popular diets: Atkins, The Zone, Weight Watchers, and Ornish. These diets were chosen because they represent the four current weight-loss trends: low carb, fewer carbs/more protein, calorie counting, and very low fat. After one year, the volunteers on the Atkins diet had lost an average of four pounds, and those on the other three diets had lost an average of five pounds. The dropout rate on all the diets was about 50 percent.

The biggest problem with just eating less, especially on a crash diet, is hunger. Yes, weight peels off at first, and that's usually very exciting. Who doesn't want immediate results? But then, very quickly, you hit a wall. You're constantly hungry. The hunger whittles down your resolve. You get discouraged, "break" your diet, eat more, and the weight returns. Sound familiar?

And, of course, we all know that hungry people are not happy peo-ple. When you put yourself on a restricted diet, you deny yourself the comfort and delight of food. You can't eat fewer calories for long unless you generally feel satisfied and happy.

The last time I checked, there were only smiling faces walking the beautiful grounds of the Pritikin Center. No disgruntled, hungry, dis-couraged dieters here! With nearly three decades of research and suc-cess under our belts, we know full well that the number-one surefire can't-fail secret to losing weight is to ditch the fad diets once and for all and commit to living a better, more healthful lifestyle on every level.

THE FUNDAMENTALS OF WEIGHT LOSS

The guiding principle of weight loss is surprisingly simple: it comes down to the age-old formula of burning more calories than you consume.

Calories aren't the enemy. A calorie is just a unit of energy—something many of you might recall from your days of middle-school science. A calorie is the measurement of energy required to raise the temperature of one kilogram of water by one degree Celsius. We need calories to keep us warm, fuel our body's chemical reactions, and enable us to perform physical activities. Even thinking requires calories. (I know what you're thinking, and the answer is no—eating more does not make you a genius and thinking more or harder will not make you thin.) What we don't need are *excess* calories, because the calories you consume above and beyond what you burn on a daily basis are converted into fat.

Ask Dr. Bob

Question: Is it better to eat fewer calories or to burn more calories?

Answer: In the world of obesity, they are equal. A calorie not eaten is the same as a calorie burned; your hips and belly don't care which one it is. In the world of health, however, breaking science suggests that it is better not to eat the excess calories in the first place.

Weight-Loss Arithmetic

Understanding the math of weight gain is wonderful, because it explains how we actually gain weight and what we need to do in order to lose it.

Let's start with the two basic rules of weight loss:

1. 3,500 excess calories eaten = about 1 pound of fat weight gained (you may gain some water weight that accompanies overeating, as well)
2. 1 mile walked = about 100 calories burned

So you see, it isn't difficult to lose weight (it is, however, difficult to become rail-thin by next Thursday). Say you've had a 50-pound excess weight gain. That would represent 175,000 excess calories that you ate in the past. If you stopped eating completely, it would take about three months to lose the 50 pounds. (Do not even *think* about attempting this; in reality, you would be so hungry by the second day that you would eat everything in sight.) Alternatively, you could walk or jog an additional 1,750 miles, or halfway across the country. If you jogged a 26-mile marathon every day for the next two months, you would lose the 50 pounds, but only if you didn't increase what you ate. Since starvation diets and daily marathons are not realistic, clearly a more tempered approach to trimming and expending calories is the way to go.

The biggest fallacy about obese people is that they eat a whole lot more than thin people. This is not true. Most of us eat about 750,000 calories each year. Obese people may eat as little as only 10 percent more than thin people, but that 10 percent can make a big difference. Adding even a few extra calories each day packs on the pounds faster than you might think. Therefore it's not what happens every few weeks or months that matters as much as what your typical daily choices are.

Let's suppose that your weight is stable. How much weight would you gain in a year if you added just one 100-calorie cookie to your diet? The astounding answer is about 10 pounds. Can one cookie more per day really make you obese? Again, let's take pen to paper. According to the formula, 100 calories more per day is about one pound more per month. Multiply that pound by 12 months and you will gain about 10 pounds; in five years it's 50 pounds! Now you're obese, and the cause is one measly cookie a day. You would gain only 25 pounds or so if you continued your usual physical activity, because your larger body would need more calories to function. Unfortunately, though, physical activity generally diminishes as we gain weight. If that happens, you'd gain the full 50 pounds . . . all from adding one innocent medium-sized cookie every day!

Now let's reverse this theoretical cookie experiment. If your weight was now stable (i.e. you were not currently gaining weight), how much less would you weigh in five years if you ate one fewer 100-calorie cookie? It's of course the same 25 to 50 pounds. I'm not trying to fool you; you really can lose 50 pounds without changing anything other than one 100-calorie cookie per day—but it would take five years.

The key concept to remember is that, generally speaking, 100 fewer calories per day is 10 pounds lighter in a year. What is 100 calories? My mental image for 100 calories is one slice of bread, one package of 100-calorie snack food, one pat of butter, one eight-ounce glass of a regular soft drink, or one medium-sized cookie/two small cookies.

Of course you can lose the 50 pounds faster with a little more effort. You probably could eat two fewer cookies per day, or their equivalent 200 calories, and still feel very satisfied with all the other food you're eating, especially if those 200 calories came from calorie-dense foods like pure fats (butter and oils), chips, cheeses, and yes, cookies. That would be about 10 percent fewer calories than you are currently eating. You would lose as much as 50 pounds in half the time, or two and a half years.

Now let's look at the second equation, the amount of calories expended. I know that you, like me, are probably willing to take only a cookie or two out of your diet. We all like cookies!

Burning Fat with Sneakers

There are, much to my regret, no foods that burn calories. However, if you walk an additional two miles each day (3,500 to 4,000 steps), you will burn about another 200 calories per day. Walking quickly or uphill burns even more calories. Everyone is individual, but there are many guests who have lost 50 pounds or more in a year following the Pritikin Program of eating less and walking more. In a recent weight-loss study done by Brown University, women who dieted and walked 10 miles more per week lost 30 pounds in a year, while the women who only dieted lost 13 pounds. This 17-pound additional weight loss is almost exactly what would be predicted by the 100 calories burned per mile rule.

Right now, you probably walk 4,000 to 7,000 steps a day. One of the first things I instruct all my patients to do is to buy a pedometer and start logging their steps, then increase the amount they walk each day by 3,500 to 4,000 steps, or about two miles. More walking does not take too much time, but it does take a change in how you approach everyday activities. You'll learn more about how to incorporate more walking into your daily life in Chapter 10, but in the meantime, here are a few easy ways to start logging more steps:

- Park as far away from where you are going as possible. The time you spend circling around looking for a close-in parking space can easily be converted into walking.
- Get a dog, and let it walk you.
- Walk on the golf course. You'll feel more relaxed when you flub a shot.
- Take the stairs rather than the escalator or elevator.
- Make it a practice to enjoy a 15- to 20-minute walk in the morning or after dinner. Savor it as precious alone time, or quality time with a friend or family member; the emotional nourishment you'll get from it doubles the benefit.
- If you're traveling, take a lap or two around the airport or hotel. I've been spotted in many a hotel doing short, easy laps up and down the hallways.

The Hunger Factor

One of the biggest concerns people have when embarking on a weight-loss plan is that they will be hungry. But hunger is never a problem on the Pritikin Program. We make sure of that.

Breathing, thirst, and hunger are the three most powerful survival instincts. No one voluntarily goes hungry for very long, which is why successful weight loss depends on understanding how to satisfy this basic instinct. The cycle of hunger/satiety depends on the dance between several important hormones such as *ghrelin* and *cholecystokinin*.

Ghrelin is a key chemical messenger, or hormone, in the hunger story. Ghrelin is made by the stomach and acts on the hypothalamic region of the brain. The hypothalamus receives many different body signals about nutrition and digestion and orchestrates the appropriate hunger and satiety responses. Ghrelin levels rise sharply when we are hungry and fall immediately after we eat. Prolonged calorie restriction increases ghrelin levels, which points to a likely reason why crash diets do not work. Sooner or later, you get so hungry that you eat everything in sight.

Hunger is quenched when your stomach is distended and empties. Stomach distension—or stretching—decreases ghrelin production and signals your brain that you have eaten enough. After a meal, your stomach secretes digestive juices, further distending it. Technically, the satiety signals do not reach your brain until about 20 minutes after you have begun eating.

Cholecystokinin is a hormone made by the small intestine when the stomach empties. Satiety occurs when ghrelin levels fall and cholecystokinin levels rise. Similar to stomach distention, stomach emptying takes time. This is why we feel more satisfied a little while after we finish eating. Remember last Thanksgiving? You knew you ate too much, but you didn't feel really stuffed until a little later. Belch!

There are a few other hormones that make us feel satisfied, including one called *leptin*. Leptin is made by fat cells that are stuffed full, and it is responsible for decreasing our appetite. Mice—and even humans—without leptin grow enormously obese. Highly processed high-fructose corn syrup, found in most regular soft drinks and many sugary snack foods, does not increase leptin, hence after consuming it you don't feel full and just keep on eating. Obese people have high leptin levels but have developed leptin resistance because of their excess weight.

With all of these built-in hunger and satiety controls, why do people become obese? Because we eat refined (processed), calorie-dense foods that neither stretch our stomachs nor produce satiety, and we consume sugar-dense foods and beverages that provide little satiety per calorie. Mix these factors together with inexpensive, ubiquitous, highly varied, artificially tasty, and pervasively advertised food, and you have near-worldwide gluttony.

MAKING SMART FOOD CHOICES

How can you fight back and avoid or reverse obesity? By learning that not all foods are created equal, and making choices that send the right signals to your hormones so you feel full and satisfied. It all comes down to understanding the difference between foods that are "calorie-dense" and "calorie-light."

Stomach stretch receptors tell us that we've eaten enough after ingesting meals of a certain size and weight. Calories don't count to the stretch receptors; they respond to volume. Part of losing weight and feeling full is expanding your stomach with more food but fewer calories. In other words, we need to choose more calorie-light foods and cut back on the calorie-dense foods. Ideally, you want to average less than about 500 calories per pound.

Foods that contain a lot of water and fiber are calorie-light. Fruits, vegetables, cooked high-fiber grains, and soups are good examples of calorie-light foods. In general, foods with less than one calorie per gram are calorie-light. That translates to less than about 500 calories per pound.

Calorie-light foods are rarely fast foods, which are generally calorie-dense. A hearty bean soup may sound fattening, but with 240 calories per pound of the bean soup, it is really calorie-light. On the other hand, graham crackers are a whopping 1,900 calories per pound, and are calorie-packed. Think about that: one ounce of graham crackers (which is the same as ¹⁄₁₆ pound of graham crackers, which is about four little graham crackers) contains the same number of calories as a half pound of bean soup. Which do you think is the better choice to signal your stretch receptors and make you feel satisfied and full?

You can easily ruin calorie-light foods by turning them into calorie-dense foods: just add pure fat, refined flour, and/or sugar. A great example is the potato. At 490 calories per pound, a baked potato is a pretty good food, but fry it or load it with butter, cheese, and bacon bits and you're on your way to obesity. Pringles have about 2,900 calories per pound (six calories per gram). If you can't get fat eating Pringles, you gave it your best shot. French fries contain about 1,450 calories per pound and, sadly, are America's favorite vegetable. French fries rank as the second-favorite food of American men (the first being hamburgers), but they top the list for women. My wife often tells me that women are smarter than men. Ha!

Calculating Calorie Density

As you can see from the Calorie Density table on page 56, vegetables have very few calories per pound: a pound of vegetables adds up to, at most, 195 calories. It's one whole pound of food—a lot of volume, but not a lot of calories. That's critical to emphasize, because the storage capacity of your stomach is only about two to three pounds, and your stomach really doesn't care whether you eat 500 calories to fill it up or 5,000. Once it's filled to capacity and its stretch receptors have alerted you that it's full, you're pretty much done eating.

To illustrate, imagine that your stomach is a goldfish bowl that holds about two pounds of food. First, fill your goldfish bowl with peanuts. Well, your bowl's full, but you've just eaten—gulp!—more than 5,000 calories. Now, empty the bowl and fill it up with sliced bananas. This time about 700 calories—just *one-seventh* of the calories—fill up the bowl. Big difference. If you filled half the bowl with peanuts and half with bananas, the calorie intake would be the average of the two—still better than it was with just the nuts.

A man feels satisfied with about four pounds of food a day, a woman with about three pounds. So, if you are filling your stomach up with a lot of the right calorie-light foods (say, foods at 450 calories per pound), you will fill your stomach and be satisfied with fewer calories. All without ever feeling hungry and without ever having counted calories.

Balancing Calorie-Dense and Calorie-Light Foods

A bowl of shredded wheat is a terrific breakfast, especially if topped with fruit and mixed with skim milk. At 1,600 calories per pound (100 calories per ounce), however, how can shredded wheat be considered a weight-reducing breakfast? The answer lies in realizing that that bowl contains a mixture of calorie-dense and calorie-light foods that together create a *calorie-light combination.*

Here's how that works: shredded wheat alone weighs in at 1,600 calories per pound, or 100 calories per ounce. If you're having dry cereal like shredded wheat, pour less cereal in your bowl and fill half your bowl with lots of fruit (300 calories per pound). The result? A lower calorie density. The fruit fills you up and keeps you from eating too much of the calorie-concentrated cereal. Your calorie intake is now averaging about 950 calories per pound.

Create a calorie-light combination that's even better by combining a hot cereal like oatmeal (280 calories per pound) with fruit (300 calories per pound). You're now down to a hearty, filling, tasty breakfast that's just 290 calories per pound, about *one-third* the calorie density of a dry-cereal breakfast. The key is to eat enough calorie-light foods that are great for health and satiety to balance the calorie-dense ones that make us fat.

I know what you're thinking: Why not just drink a lot of water? Wouldn't water fill me up? Not really. While it's true that loading up with water means you have a full stomach with zero calories, the water doesn't *stay* in your stomach very long. That's right—you're running to the bathroom before you know it. And soon after, you're hungry.

By contrast, water that has been integrated into food via the *cooking process* (like oats cooked with water or pasta boiled with water) *does* add long-term satisfaction, and increases the weight and volume of the food in your fishbowl belly without adding calories.

Here are some examples of foods and how they measure on the calorie-density scale.

Foods and Their Calorie Density (total number of calories, per pound)

Food	Calories per pound
Vegetables	65 to 195
Fresh fruits	135 to 420
Nonfat dairy foods	180 to 450
Potatoes, pastas, brown rice, sweet potatoes, corn, hot cereals	280 to 650
Legumes: peas and beans, such as pinto, garbanzo, black, and lentil beans	400 to 750
Seafood, lean poultry, lean red meat	400 to 870
Dried fruit, jams, fat-free muffins, and all breads, including sourdough rolls, bagels, pita breads, and baguettes	1,200 to 1,400
Dry cereal, pretzels, fat-free cookies, fat-free potato chips	1,600 to 1,780
Regular salad dressing	1,800 to 2,000
Chocolate bars, croissants, doughnuts	2,200 to 2,500
Nuts, regular potato chips	2,500 to 3,000
Butter, margarine	3,200
Olive oil, corn oil, lard	4,010

Calorie-light foods	Calories per pound	Calorie-light foods	Calories per pound
Lettuce	65	Onions	155
Cucumbers	70	Tofu, light	190
Tomatoes	90	Carrots	195
Spinach	100	Oranges	210
Mushrooms	115	Nectarines	220
Broccoli	130	Apples	270
Berries	140	Pears	270
Cantaloupe	140	Oatmeal	280
Grapefruit	150	Kiwi	280
Watermelon	150	Grapes	300

Calorie-moderate foods	Calories per pound	Calorie-dense foods	Calories per pound
Bananas	420	Pizza, cheese	1,010
Sour cream, fat free	425	Dried apricots	1,080
Cottage cheese/no fat	430	Ground beef (lean)	1,235
Crab, cooked	460	Bread	1,240
Cod, cooked	480	Bagels	1,270
Potatoes, baked	490	Chicken nuggets	1,340
Corn, cooked without fat	490	French fries	1,450
Rice, brown, cooked	500	Sausage, Italian	1,470
Beans, pinto, cooked without fat	510	Cream cheese	1,580
		Swiss cheese	1,700
Couscous, cooked	510	Popcorn, plain	1,730
Peas, cooked without fat	520	Cornflakes	1,770
Yams, baked	525	Pretzels	1,770
Veggie burgers	600	Cheerios	1,780
Pasta, cooked	630	Cheddar cheese	1,820
Shrimp, boiled	630	Carrot cake	1,850
Salmon, poached	660	Goldfish snacks	2,120
Chicken breast, without skin	750	Granola bar	2,140
		Chocolate chip cookies	2,140
Pork tenderloin	750	M&M's candy	2,270
Ground turkey, lean	780	Tortilla chips	2,400
Avocados	800	Peanuts	2,640
Hummus	810	Butter, margarine	3,200
Bison	860	Oils	4,010

Calories Count, but Don't Count Calories

We need to eat only about 12 calories per pound of body weight per day to maintain a constant weight if we are not very physically active. So, to translate, if you're five feet six inches tall and 140 pounds, 1,700 calories per day is about right for you. At six feet tall and 170 pounds, 2,000 is sufficient. Most moderately active Americans should average somewhere between 1,900 and 2,000 calories per day.

Now, forget what I just told you. Yes, that's right; having said all that, I don't want you to count calories. It is too difficult, especially if, like many of us, you eat out a lot. Besides, you are going to cheat; you won't count all the calories that you eat. In several careful food diary trials, obese volunteers omitted 400 to 1,000 calories they consumed each day, or about one-third of their total caloric intake. Asking overweight people how much they eat is like asking prison inmates whether they are guilty. That's what scales are for, whether they are the justice or bathroom variety.

What happens is something like this: You have a "snack" at midnight. Since you have already finished the present day's calorie log, you won't add it to that page. You haven't yet started the next day's log, so the snack won't go on that page, either. The snack just didn't happen, according to your food log.

Or maybe you'll carefully write down that you had a 110-calorie soft drink. The problem is that the 16 ounces you just drank are really two 110-calorie portions. One of the most important pieces of information listed on nutrition labels is portion size. One 16-ounce soft drink is two portions, containing 110 calories each. In reality, you consumed 220 calories, not 110.

One bagel is actually two portions; a package of two medium cookies is two portions, and so on. The food industry is contributing to our obesity by packaging two or more portions of a food meant to be eaten by one person. This is deceptive labeling. Again, it's not necessarily a conspiracy on their part; it's just business. It's up to us to learn to read the labels more carefully (you'll learn more about this in Part Five).

In any case, we don't want you to count calories. We want you to eat more calorie-light food and less calorie-dense food, period.

You might be wondering, if you don't count calories, how are you going to know how much to eat? Simple. Although dieters fib, scales don't. Weigh yourself regularly. You have cut down sufficiently if you are losing a pound or two every month. If you're not losing weight, it's time to cut out more French fries.

Why the Glycemic Index Doesn't Matter

In the diet book wars of recent years, the glycemic index has aroused a loud rallying cry. Some books even tell you to avoid eating raw carrots because they have a high glycemic index. To us at Pritikin, advice like this is hogwash. Don't eat *carrots*?!?

The glycemic index is a measure of how much a specific food raises blood sugar. The index arbitrarily sets white bread to a value of 100. A baked white potato has a high glycemic index of 85 and an apple a low value of 39. In theory, high glycemic index foods spike your blood sugar, which then falls due to insulin release. With low blood sugar, you become hungry again.

Choosing foods by their glycemic index is nutritional nonsense. Why? The glycemic index measures blood sugar increases after eating an amount of the specific food containing 50 grams (about two ounces) of carbohydrate. Fifty grams of carbohydrate is contained in two ounces of sugar-dense foods like junk food, but also in pounds of low-carbohydrate foods like carrots. Carrots have a high glycemic index but very little carbohydrate. You'd have to eat more than a pound of carrots to spike your blood sugar as high as the glycemic index warns, and you'd have to eat more than 19 pounds of raw carrots to gain one pound of weight. Beware books recommending that carrots, with their high glycemic index, make you fat.

A food's glycemic index can also vary significantly depending on how it's actually eaten. Adding fat and/or protein generally lowers its glycemic index because it slows absorption of the sugar. Adding dollops of sour cream to a baked potato actually lowers its index, but clearly doesn't make it a healthier, waist-slimming food.

A recent analysis from the Nurses' Health Study of 82,000 women suggested that high-carbohydrate diets, loaded with lots of sugar and refined carbs, are associated with more heart disease. In the same study, high-carbohydrate, high fruit and vegetable diets had less heart disease. This observation underscores the stupidity of simply characterizing a high- or low-carb diet as healthy. Unlike the glycemic index, focusing on unrefined, low-calorie-dense foods works all of the time.

Forget the "glycemic load" as well. This is another measure that takes the amount of carbohydrate in a portion into consideration. In no way are French fries with lower glycemic loads better foods than baked potatoes (without the sour cream).

What Does the Research Have to Say?

At Pritikin, we have the same general opinion of this tool as the expert committee of scientists appointed by the U.S. Department of Agriculture to develop the 2005 U.S. Dietary Guidelines. The committee wrote: "Current evidence suggests that the glycemic index and/or glycemic load are of little utility for providing dietary guidance for Americans."

Recently published, also, was an exhaustive review of 140 studies on carbohydrate intake and body-mass index. It found there was no connection between the glycemic index and BMI. The University of Virginia scientists concluded that people should focus on fiber-rich carbohydrates and not worry about the glycemic index or eating too many carbohydrates.

Refined and Processed Foods

One of the easiest ways to ruin a perfectly healthy food is to process or "refine" it. Refined food is an oxymoron. Refining food generally reduces its water and fiber content, which in turn reduce bulk, chewing time, and satiety. Think how quickly a handful of potato chips goes down compared to a big baked potato, though they're similar in calorie content. In the refining process, key nutrients are usually lost as well. What's left is calorie-dense, nutritionally destitute junk food in a gaudy, misleadingly labeled package. Refined? I don't think so. Refined eaters don't eat refined foods.

How can you recognize refined and overly processed food when you see it? Simple; it looks nothing like anything that came out of the earth. The farther we get from what nature grows (apple juice instead of an apple, French fries instead of a baked potato), the worse off we tend to be.

By stripping foods of their nutritional riches, we humans have regressed healthwise. Our insides haven't changed much in the last 20,000 years, but our food preparation practices surely have. What our ancestors ate thousands of years ago is what our bodies are designed to eat now. On the outside we may be wearing Nikes and Armani, but on the inside we're still hunter-gatherers that thrive on fiber-rich, straight-from-the-earth fuel. Ironically, it's the "unrefined" rural countries still eating the diets of their ancestors that enjoy the lowest rates of obesity, diabetes, high blood pressure, and heart disease. We "refined" nations, on the other hand, are getting fatter and sicker.

Satiety Index (aka "What to Eat So You Feel Full")

Satiety is the opposite of hunger. The more satisfied, or satiated, you feel after eating a meal or snack, the greater the satiety value of that meal or snack. Satiety is also a measure of how long it takes for you to become hungry again after eating a meal. A high-satiety meal will make you feel very full initially and will also stave off hunger for quite a few hours after you've eaten. A low-satiety meal or snack does not leave you satisfied. You're still hungry, on the hunt for more to eat.

Of course, plenty of calorie-dense foods, in large amounts, have a high level of satiety. Jars of cashews and bags of Doritos will keep you full and satisfied all day long. But all those calories, as you well know, put on weight, too. Lots of weight. There are, however, many high-satiety foods that *don't* flood your body with excess calories.

In the satiety index, foods are rated by how much food people ate after consuming them to satisfy their hunger. All are compared to white bread, which again is ranked as "100." Research showed that boiled potatoes were the foods with the highest satiety rating: 323. Croissants were the lowest, at 47. This means that, per calorie, it would take more than *six times* the amount of croissants to give you the same level of satiety as potatoes. You may be very surprised to learn that French fries are much less satisfying than boiled potatoes. Whole-grain bread was found to be 50 percent more filling than white bread. Not surprisingly, among the least filling foods are cakes, doughnuts, and cookies (all high in fat, sugar, and refined carbohydrates).

The following is a list of common foods and how they rank on the satiety index. (Tip: If you want to lose weight, avoid the LOWER numbers! The lower the number, the lower the satiety level of that particular food.)

Bakery Products	
Croissants	47
Cake	65
Doughnuts	68
Cookies	120
Crackers	127

Snacks and Confectionary	
Mars candy bar	70
Peanuts	84
Yogurt	88
Crisps	91
Ice cream	96
Jelly beans	118
Popcorn	154

Breakfast Cereals	
Muesli	100
Sustain	112
Special K	116
Cornflakes	118
Honey Smacks	132
All-Bran	151
Porridge/Oatmeal	209

Carbohydrate-rich Foods	
White bread	100
French fries	116
White pasta	119
Brown rice	132
White rice	138
Whole-grain bread	154
Whole-meal bread	157
Brown pasta	188
Potatoes	323

Protein-Rich Foods	
Lentils	133
Cheese	146
Eggs	150
Baked beans	168
Beef	176

Fruits	
Bananas	118
Grapes	162
Apples	197
Oranges	202

Table adapted from S.H.A. Holt, J.C. Brand Miller, P. Petocz, and E. Farmakalidis, "A Satiety Index of Common Foods," *European Journal of Clinical Nutrition* 49(9): 675–90.

The Pleasure of Dining

Think about treating yourself to a good meal at a fancy restaurant where the courses are served separately, deliberately, and slowly. Each dish is presented beautifully so that it is a feast for all your senses. You start with a small appetizer, followed after some time by a soup or salad. Internally, all the right things are happening: your stomach gets distended and perhaps has started to empty. Ghrelin levels have begun to fall, cholecystokinin levels are rising, and satiety signals are going to your brain. By the time the entrée arrives, you are not too hungry and the food portions look pretty large. You could eat half the entrée and feel more than satisfied.

That is exactly what I'm begging you to do. Take that hand off your fork and slowly back away from the table as satiety sets in. Take the rest home. Wait until later before even considering dessert.

Interestingly, though you *could* back away, you don't. Why? After all, you paid for it, it tastes good, you had a rough day, and your parents trained you to finish your plate, no matter what. Your emotions and habits are overriding your basic biological instincts. Obesity is truly complex.

If this were a fast-food restaurant, you wouldn't have a chance to make the observation that you really aren't hungry before wolfing down the last bite. Eating fast food is the culinary equivalent of a car crash. It just happens too fast. Fine dining experiences provide important lessons about how we can learn to slow down and enjoy our food, so that we ultimately eat better—but far fewer—calories.

Ask Dr. Bob

Question: How do I know how much to eat?

Answer: Eat only when you are hungry and STOP the instant you're comfortable. Anything beyond that and you'll feel stuffed.

Fat Calories versus Carbohydrate Calories

There's been so much hype and hoopla over the past few years about diets that are "low-fat" and "low-carb" that it's no wonder Americans are thoroughly confused about losing weight. There are literally tens of thousands of different diet books out there, proving only that there are a whole lot of fat people willing to spend a whole lot of money on losing weight.

So, should you cut out fat, or carbohydrates? Do you really have to give up eating carrots and bananas? (The quick answer to this is that anyone who suggests so is a nutritional idiot.) Are "low-fat" snack foods better for you? (Short answer: not necessarily.) The way we distill the truth of the whole low-fat versus low-carb debate is by explaining that it isn't about cutting out either. It's about eating healthy foods and following the Pritikin principle of calorie density. In other words, get rid of:

- Calorie-dense fatty foods loaded with saturated and trans fats
- Calorie-dense, highly refined and processed foods with sugar and white flour
- Foods that are loaded with both, such as ice cream, donuts, pastries, pies, and cakes, and many kids' cereals

Dr. Robert Atkins popularized a very low carbohydrate approach to weight loss several years back. At the other end of the spectrum, and much healthier, is a very low-fat, almost vegetarian diet. We at the Pritikin Longevity Center do not focus on individual food components such as carbs or fat. Rather, our focus is on healthy, nutrient-rich foods. The Pritikin Program turns out to be moderately low in fat as a *natural consequence of its emphasis on eating a lot of really healthy food.* Once you get in the habit of eating more salads, soups, fruits, fish, and whole-grain dishes, you are just not going to have enough room for fat-packed double cheeseburgers or a craving for overly sugary low-fat cookies. Nor will you be hungry, even though you are eating fewer calories. Your stomach will be content and your blood sugar will be stable. Over time, your cravings for greasy or sickly sweet foods melt away.

Making Sense of Low-Carbohydrate Diets

A low-carbohydrate diet really means a high-fat diet. To describe any low-carbohydrate diet as a high-protein diet is nonsense. High-protein foods like meat and cheese usually contain most of their calories as fat. Even high-protein tofu contains a lot of fat (about 47 percent of total calories). Fortunately, it also contains a lot of water and is generally calorie-light.

In several ways, the popular low-carbohydrate diets out there today are doing us harm. We Americans eat about 20 percent of our calories as protein; we do not need to eat more, as high-protein diets injure the kidneys.

Muscles can be fueled by either fat or sugar, but the brain runs only on sugar. We need about three ounces of carbohydrates daily to fuel our brains. Without enough carbohydrates, we use up our glycogen stores and then break down fat and muscle. Breaking down fat may be desirable, but breaking down muscle is a disaster.

Observing different cultures tells us a lot about healthy eating. Most long-living cultures, such as the Japanese and Mediterraneans, eat ample amounts of carbohydrates from whole grains, fruits, and vegetables. The Japanese eat a lot of rice and live about five years longer than we do. The Andorrans live even longer on a Mediterranean diet of whole-grain bread, pasta, fruits, vegetables, and seafood. The principality of Andorra is tucked between France and Spain. The great longevity of the Mediterranean and Pacific Rim regions eating high-carbohydrates diets is the strongest evidence against the idea that all carbohydrates are evil.

Why, then, are low-carbohydrate diets so popular? Because low-carb diets shed pounds in the short term, and instant gratification is very alluring when it comes to weight loss. Who wouldn't want to drop a dress or pant size in two weeks? The results are fleeting, though. Most of the weight lost short term on a low-carbohydrate diet is water, not fat, and it eventually comes back once we start eating normally again. For all the reasons we already discussed, our bodies need carbohydrates to function properly (for energy, brain fuel, muscle function, and so on). Severely restricting carbohydrate-containing foods restricts our choices, which is a recipe for dissatisfaction—remember, emotional fulfillment is a major component to overall wellness. An eating plan needs to complement and enhance our lifestyle, not cripple it, if we're to sustain it long term.

To be fair to low-carbohydrate diets, there is one sensible part that we applaud them for: advising people to eat less refined, processed foods. That's *always* a good thing. For years, the team at Pritikin has advocated replacing the mounds of sugar and white flour Americans eat daily with fruits, vegetables, whole grains, and lean protein like fish.

Making Sense Out of Low-fat Diets

The 1970s saw the beginning of the advice to cut fat consumption to reduce heart disease in America. In its intent, that advice was sound, but the result has instead turned out to be a health disaster. In response to the call to reduce fat, our food industry invented countless highly processed "low-fat" foods loaded with sugar, refined grains, trans fats, and salt. "Diet" versions of everything, from cookies to ice cream to packaged TV dinners, swept the nation. Unfortunately, these items usually have as many calories as the original high-fat foods they were designed to replace. As a percentage of total calories, America's direct fat consumption did decrease about 5 percent during the past two decades. However, since our total calorie intake increased, *total fat consumption has actually increased.* Yes, that's right: though America was on a "low-fat" diet, Americans actually ate *more fat.* We won the fat-content battle, so to speak, but lost the obesity war.

At the same time, we are annually eating 30 more pounds of sugar per person. Adults now eat 150 pounds of sugar per year; teenagers eat 250 pounds. The average American family with two teenagers eats 800 pounds of sugar annually. That's almost half a ton! Not surprisingly, obesity and diabetes have dramatically increased over the past three decades, especially in youngsters.

The Sugar/Fat Sleight of Hand

We now eat so much sugar that it only appears that we are eating less fat. Here's how adding sugar "reduces" the percentage of fat in foods:

An eight-ounce glass of whole milk gets 50 percent of its 150 calories from fat. If you add three tablespoons of fat-free but sugar-laden chocolate syrup, the total calorie content soars to 300 calories, but the milk now gets only 25 percent of its calories from fat. Yes, your chocolate milk is lower in fat percentage. Do you really believe that chocolate milk is going to help people lose weight and improve their health because its percentage of fat calories was cut in half? I don't think so.

Very low-fat diets (containing less than 10 percent of calories from fat) are based on the observation that heart disease generally parallels fat consumption. One study did show that a very low-fat diet, combined with exercise and relaxation training, actually reduced coronary artery blockage. Though consistent with the Pritikin Program, very low-fat diets take a lot of motivation for people to sustain them for very long.

The Pritikin Program, because it recommends naturally low-fat, fiber-rich foods, turns out to be a *moderately* low-fat diet (containing about 15 to 20 percent of calories from fat). The Japanese are living proof that even a moderately low-fat diet rich in fruits, vegetables, and fish reduces heart disease and extends longevity. That's not to say the Japanese diet is perfect—it contains a lot of salt—but their longevity proves they are doing something right. Pritikin is living proof, too. A five-year study following 64 men who came to Pritikin instead of undergoing coronary bypass surgery found that 80 percent never needed the surgery.

The bottom line is that neither very low-fat nor low-carbohydrate "dieting" is the single long-term solution to obesity. Calories, food constituents, exercise, and emotions all count, too.

READY, SET, GO

Okay, now you're armed with the facts and fundamentals of weight. After you check with your physician and make sure that your weight issues do not have a primary medical or psychological cause (such as low thyroid function or untreated depression), the last, and perhaps most important, step is getting into the right mind frame to set yourself up to succeed.

I have eight basic questions that I pose to all my patients who are embarking on a weight-loss plan. I tell them that if they expect to lose weight and keep it off, they need to be able to honestly answer yes to all eight.

Ask yourself:

1. Do you believe that being overweight is harming the quality of your life?
2. Do you understand how being overweight is shortening your life?
3. Do you accept that you are personally responsible for your weight and that heredity and body type are only a small part of the problem?
4. Do you understand that long-term lifestyle changes work, but that crash diets of any kind do not?
5. Are you aware—and in agreement—that weight loss will make your life goals easier, but will not make you a different person than you are right now?
6. Are you prepared to devote the time to increasing your physical activity?
7. Are you confident of reaching and maintaining a healthy weight goal?
8. Are you ready to say no to tempting treats and deal with disappointments and stress in a noncaloric fashion?

If you can truly answer yes to all eight of these questions, you're ready. Welcome to the Pritikin Program. We're glad you're here.

Setting Realistic Goals

Set a weight-loss goal for yourself that feels reasonable and sustainable. Following the 10 essentials, losing 20 pounds in one year is an easily attainable goal. Certainly, you may want or need to lose more, and that's fine. But in our culture, we're used to instant gratification, so we advise everyone who comes to Pritikin or follows the program not to set a time course for weight loss that is less than six months.

Remember, this is a new lifestyle you're adopting. You want to learn how to stay thin indefinitely, because the real goal is health, happiness, and a better quality of life.

MARGARET'S SECOND VISIT

Margaret came back a month later with a smile on her face. My nurse had already weighed her in at 167 pounds, five pounds less than a month ago. I congratulated her on her progress, and reminded her again that all diets work for a while, but that she'd need to continue making overall lifestyle changes—for good—in order to keep up the weight loss.

We talked about how Margaret had implemented the general game plan I had given her, starting with salads and soups. She was now eating a salad almost every day for lunch, topped by vinegar and a little oil that she kept in her desk drawer; she'd given up those calorie-dense packets of commercial salad dressing.

At home, she was starting dinner with a big salad or bowl of soup and cooking small portions of an entrée. Her husband had noticed that there wasn't enough entrée for seconds, but he certainly wasn't leaving the table hungry. He was fine with dropping a few pounds himself, in fact. He had never bugged her about her weight, so Margaret was surprised that he appeared quite pleased by the thought of a slimmer wife.

In restaurants, she had adopted the calorie-dense food tip that my wife taught me (you'll learn more tips like these in Part Two). Before starting to eat, she would cut off part of all calorie-packed foods she was served, put the excess on her side plate, and pepper them heavily. A few of her coworkers had even been inspired to do the same. Though she'd been tempted a few times to scrape off the pepper and eat the excess, she'd resisted. I gave her the mental picture of smokers trying to quit going through old garbage looking for butts, and she grimaced and said she would absolutely use that image in the future if she was ever tempted again!

I reinforced that I only wanted her to cut back on calorie-dense foods and that she could have all the salads, fruits, and soups she wanted. Margaret admitted she didn't feel as if she were dieting, as she had in the past, because she didn't feel deprived. That comment made me smile; successful weight loss should add to the quality of one's life, never detract from it. That's one of the biggest secrets to success.

We next talked about fast food, which, as you'll recall, was formerly a staple in Margaret's diet. She told me that she couldn't get out of her mind the study I quoted documenting that people who eat fast food two or more times per week had double the incidence of diabetes in 15 years. She had an aunt who was diabetic and didn't want to develop the disease herself. It turns out the food Margaret was now getting from the deli section of her upscale supermarket was a lot tastier and more varied than the fast food she had been eating. The salad greens were fresher, and there was a myriad of calorie-light salad toppings for lunch and healthful prepared foods for dinner. Margaret had discovered that good food really is more satisfying than junk food. The surprising bonuses were that buying it really didn't take more time, and the food was only minimally more expensive than fast food.

Margaret had discovered that she was eating about 10 grams of salt daily—much more than what is recommended. Because she understood the implications of salt on high blood pressure (which you'll learn more about in Chapter 12), she'd thrown out all the salt shakers at home and was experimenting with other seasonings. She was aghast at finding out how much salt there is in regular canned soups and how few low-sodium varieties were on the shelves. The solution for Margaret was to look for the Pritikin canned soups or other low-sodium varieties in the markets, order the frozen soups from the Pritikin website, or try the soup recipes in this book. Tasty to begin with, after a week of less salt in her diet they tasted marvelous. Moreover, she could now fully taste the nuttiness of whole-grain breads and pasta and the natural sweetness of corn on the cob and sweet potatoes. But Margaret now had a new problem: when she ate out, everything tasted too salty. I told her to give up on soups and known salty foods in restaurants and keep cooking her own soups at home.

Margaret had taken my recommendation of buying a pedometer and was also aghast that she was only walking between 3,000 and 4,000 steps a day, or about two miles. Having finally noticed that she and her husband weren't the only chubby members of her family, Margaret grabbed the family dog, Samantha, who was putting on extra pounds as well, and headed out for a 15-minute walk every morning and evening. She was delighted that her husband had started walking along with her, which gave them a chance to talk. Margaret started to feel better both healthwise and emotionally as a result.

Her daily steps now ranged between 5,000 and 5,500—a huge improvement for which I congratulated her. Margaret said that she knew she needed to get more exercise, and I referred her to some of my favorite exercise options, which you'll learn about in Part Two. I stressed that I wanted her to do only physical activities she enjoyed. I don't subscribe to "no pain, no gain." That may be true for competition, but it doesn't apply to obesity.

We then talked a little about the challenge of maintaining her weight-loss plan over the next few months. Because Margaret was losing weight for the right reason—her health—I assured her that her prognosis was good. Besides, I had two aces up my sleeve to keep her motivated. Margaret's blood pressure had already dropped from 138/86 to 130/82; thus, she had already reduced her risk of having a heart attack by 32 percent! The realization that her health was directly improved by her better lifestyle meant more than any changes in her appearance. Margaret had made a breakthrough.

I pulled out my second ace for future motivation. Margaret's original cholesterol values were marginal, at best (her LDL was 150; her HDL was 50). Now it was time to lower her bad cholesterol and raise her good cholesterol. Fueled by her early success, Margaret was up to the challenge. I told her to reread the last four of the 10 essential ingredients and see me in two months.

KEY POINTS TO REMEMBER

- If you want to lose weight and keep it off, you need to make overall lifestyle changes. Highly restrictive or crash diets simply don't work.
- Losing weight comes down to the basic formula of burning more calories than you consume.
- Adding even a few extra calories each day packs on the pounds faster than you might think.
- Walking is a great way to burn calories.
- Eating more calorie-light foods—rather than calorie-dense foods—is a key component of losing weight.
- Calories count, but don't count calories.
- Stick to whole foods rather than refined, processed foods.
- Low-fat and/or low-carb doesn't matter; nor does the "glycemic index." Weight loss is about choosing healthy foods and following the Pritikin principle of calorie density.
- Set a realistic weight-loss goal for yourself that feels reasonable and sustainable.

PART TWO

The 10 Essentials of the Pritikin Program

5

Pritikin Essential Ingredient 1: Healthy, Satisfying Eating Starts with Super Salads, Soups, Whole Grains, and Fruit

THE DINING ROOM is definitely the hub of the Pritikin Center. It's a truly beautiful space, to begin with. Floor-to-ceiling windows flood the spacious, three-tiered room with warm Florida sunshine, and the view just outside is the Center's sparkling outdoor swimming pool and waterfalls, flanked by palm trees and other tropical foliage. Beyond is the marina, with lovely docked yachts bobbing in the turquoise Intracoastal Waterway.

The energy inside is as uplifting as the scenery outside. Lunch is a very joyful time, because many of the guests have just come from exercise class. Their faces are flushed a wonderfully rosy color, and they're jubilant because each day they're seeing progress they never thought possible. It sounds much more like a student center at a university than a health resort. There's a lot of laughing and shouting, "Look at my new biceps!"

The salad bar is the place to be, because it's a colorful combination of about two dozen different selections: sliced red and yellow tomatoes so rich in color that they look like tomatoes our great-grandmothers grew in their gardens, exotic ingredients like jicama and roasted garlic, several varieties of beans, baby spinach, roasted corn kernels, beets, Asian greens—it's incredible. There is a soup bar as well, where people eagerly fill steaming bowls of soups like Corn Chowder.

One of the things we observe and study at Pritikin is how thinner cultures around the world tend to eat. Many, unsurprisingly, share similar good eating practices. Smart eaters dine in pleasant, uplifting surroundings. They eat slowly, enjoying their food. They start meals with filling, calorie-light foods like delicious soups and colorful, fresh salads, enjoy delicious whole grains, and don't waste calories on high-sugar beverages. They eat a lot of fruit, vegetables, whole grains, and fish. They enjoy the company of the people with whom they eat, not just the food. Sound familiar?

The first essential ingredient of the Pritikin Program focuses on the healthiest, most satisfying foods to eat that will maximize weight loss, beginning with a cornerstone of our program: *Start each meal with a super salad or soup and finish with fruit.* This is the key to eating fewer calories throughout your day without hunger. Plus, fruits and vegetables effectively lower blood pressure and supply complex nutrients that increase the production of nitric oxide. They are generally low in saturated fat and high in fiber, and displace calorie-dense foods from our diet.

Starting your meal with a good-sized salad and/or bowl of soup makes it easy to reduce your caloric intake in the main dish, because you already feel partially full. You've nourished yourself with calorie-light, healthy food, and thus won't be tempted to wolf down huge portions of calorie-dense food.

Better yet, build an entrée-size salad as your meal. Just a green salad alone has never been enough of a meal for me, but salads topped with some lean protein such as beans, poultry, or tuna fish (sans mayo) are very satisfying. My wife and I frequently eat dinner that way. If you're afraid of getting hungry, just add more greens, vegetables, or beans. Beans especially are loaded with fiber, so they will satisfy your appetite for a long time.

Super-sizing actually makes good sense when applied to salads. As I said earlier, we like to joke that the salad bowls at Pritikin are so big that they have a diving board on one end. When it comes to fresh greens, colorful veggies, and calorie-light toppings (such as beans), there's no such thing as too much. Try eating a salad for lunch rather than a sandwich. Again, I don't mean a little side salad: I mean a heaping plate from the salad bar or an entrée-sized specialty salad. Start with a big plate or bowl and pile on the greens. Next, add lots of colorful veggies: bell peppers, tomatoes, shredded carrots, or purple cabbage—whatever you like most. You don't have to forgo your favorite sandwich fillings, either, especially if they are white-meat turkey and chicken or tuna. Simply throw away the bread, cheese, and egg yolks and put the fillings on top of your masterpiece instead. You've just created your own version of a chef's salad.

If your meal consists of more than a big salad, be sure to start it with a salad—or, for variety, soup—*every time.* You can substitute a big bowl of soup (homemade or low-sodium, not store-bought salt licks!) for the side salad, or have some of each. Most soups, except very rich, creamy soups, are relatively low in calories. Unfortunately, many soups, as you already know, contain a lot of salt. Choose lower-salt soups, like our recipes in Part Three. You'll also find Pritikin soups and salad dressings at many supermarkets and health food stores, and at the store at pritikin .com. Between the salad and/or the soup, you'll very soon find your appetite for heaping entrée portions a thing of the past.

Make it a practice to finish lunch and/or dinner with fruit rather than a dessert. Anytime you make that substitution, you'll have saved yourself from eating a whole bunch of fattening calories, not to mention that fruit is very sweet and satisfying.

The Proof Is in the Produce

Our recommendation to eat more fruits and vegetables is based on solid research. In the famous Lyon and Indo-Mediterranean Diet Studies, eating more fruits and vegetables, along with other healthy changes, was shown to reduce death and cardiovascular events by 50 to 60 percent.

CASE STUDY: AMY

Amy is a charming, nearly 70-year-old avid gardener. Normally very active, she came to see me almost two years ago because of chest pain. Fortunately, it turned out not to be heart disease, but her blood pressure and cholesterol were elevated. She was five foot five and 165 pounds at that time, so we decided that losing weight was in order. We set a realistic goal for her of 20 pounds.

Amy and her husband were eating traditional American dinners of meat and potatoes. They both liked salads, but like many people, they thought of them as a "side," not as a meal. After reading an early draft of this book, she realized that she needed to switch from heavy dinners to great big salads, topped with smaller portions of fish or chicken. She lost 20 pounds in a year, and now she has the blood pressure and cholesterol of a teenager. By the way, her husband's cholesterol is also now well controlled.

I look forward to Amy's visits. We trade stories of our wonderful grandchildren, and she smiles brightly as she tells me that her garden has never looked better.

UNDRESSING YOUR SALAD

Substituting a salad for a sandwich at lunch works only if you don't drown the salad in dressing. Salad dressings often contain more than 100 calories per tablespoon. A commercial package of salad dressing contains 200 to 300 calories, which is more than the two slices of bread you just passed up. Most restaurants give you two packages worth of salad dressing, or 400 to 600 calories. The salad bar at the hospital where I practice has 2-ounce cups for dressing; every day, I watch people fill up at least one cup, if not two, for their salads. Two 2-ounce cups equals eight tablespoons—which comes to a whopping 1,000 calories. These people might as well be over on the other side of the cafeteria getting a cheeseburger and French fries, which has roughly the same number of calories.

Most commercial fat-free dressings aren't the best choice, either, since they often are loaded with salt and sugar. Calorie-free dressings are okay for weight loss, but truthfully, they don't taste very good to me! I prefer lemon juice, balsamic vinegar alone, or vinegar plus a small amount of olive, canola, or walnut oil. Any of these are fresh, tasty, low-calorie dressings that will not destroy your salad. (Please note: if you go with oil and vinegar, go easy on the oil, because each tablespoon packs 128 calories.) There are also a lot of good suggestions for salad dressings in the recipe section in Part Three.

One of the best ways we teach people to "undress" their salad is to leave the dressing on the side and simply stick their fork into it before they spear each bite of salad. You'll still get the taste of the dressing without drowning your salad in unnecessary calories.

ENJOYING FRUITS AND VEGETABLES

Which fruits and vegetables are the best choices? There really are no bad fruits or vegetables, although some offer you more benefits than others. Even romaine and the much-maligned iceberg lettuce are good choices. Calorie for calorie, they are about as nutrient rich as other lettuces. Indeed, this factoid was the catalyst for the great success of one of the Pritikin Center's most famous movie-celebrity guests, who had previously eschewed salads because he liked only iceberg and romaine lettuces, which he had heard weren't good for you. Here are some good general guidelines when it comes to choosing and preparing fruits and vegetables:

- A rough rule in choosing produce is that color counts. Deeper yellow, green, red, and purple fruits generally have more nutritional value.
- Fresh fruit is a better choice than dried, since dried fruit is several times more calorie-dense (because all the water has been squeezed out).
- While some fad diet books have demonized the white potato, there is no credible research showing it is a problem. By itself, a boiled or baked potato is just fine. The problem is that it is often fried in hydrogenated oils (French fries and chips) or topped with foods high in saturated fat, such as butter, sour cream, and cheese. Minus those, potatoes are a perfectly good choice.
- The skins of fruits and vegetables generally have high nutritional content and should be eaten, if possible.
- Cook vegetables as little as possible, and refrain from smothering them in butter or margarine. Try a small amount of canola oil instead or cook with waterless cookware (available in all cooking stores and online at pritikin.com) and see how flavorful they are when cooked in their own juices. Frying vegetables is as dumb as frying chicken. Why ruin good food?

THE FIBER ADVANTAGE

Besides being calorie-light, salads and fruit are high in fiber, which is critical to losing weight without feeling hungry. Fiber adds bulk with minimal calories, because it is mostly indigestible.

Fiber, found exclusively in grains, fruits, vegetables, legumes (beans), and nuts, comes in two forms: soluble and insoluble in water. A good example of insoluble fiber is wheat bran, the outer shell of grains that is often discarded when grains are refined or processed. Food sources of insoluble fiber include whole grains and to a lesser extent beans, vegetables, and fruits. Soluble fiber includes oat bran, psyllium, and pectin. Good food sources of soluble fiber are fruits, whole oats, beans and peas, barley, yams, sweet potatoes, new potatoes, carrots, and other vegetables. Soluble fiber has an added benefit of lowering LDL (bad) cholesterol. The rule of thumb is that roughly 10 grams of soluble fiber lowers cholesterol 5 to 10 percent.

You want to consume a minimum of 30 grams of total fiber (10 of which should be soluble fiber) daily. While we don't want you to count calories throughout the day, we do encourage our guests at Pritikin to count up their fiber grams daily. Whenever you sit down to eat, ask yourself, "How am I going to get 10 to 15 grams of fiber in each meal?"

Here are some practical, easy ways to increase your fiber intake:

- Eat more fruits and vegetables. The original fruit is always better than its juice. An unrefined and unprocessed, fiber-rich apple elevates blood sugar rather slowly; apple juice, by contrast, which is highly processed with all the fiber removed, is mostly sugar water.
- Eat more beans. They are low in calorie density and high in nutrients and fiber. All kinds of beans are good for you: kidney, garbanzo, lima, navy, and so on.
- Eat high-fiber cereals, especially those made from whole oats or whole wheat. Hot cereals such as oatmeal satisfy your hunger longer than cold cereals and are more calorie-light, because they absorb the water.
- Choose whole-grain breads and pastas over the refined, white versions.
- Leave the skin on potatoes. Sweet potatoes have more fiber than white potatoes, but both are good choices (minus the calorie-dense toppings, of course).
- Eat brown and wild rice instead of white rice. Instant rice is the worst form, because all the nutrients have been stripped away.

Three Helpful Hints When Increasing Your Fiber Intake

1. Build up the amount you add to your diet slowly (especially beans, the "musical fruit"), unless you plan to file an environmental impact statement.
2. Enzyme preparations that prevent excess gas, such as Beano, are available over the counter.
3. High-fiber foods hold on to water, reducing constipation. It's a good idea to drink more fluids as you eat more fiber-rich foods to promote this beneficial effect.

It's easy to remember the five best natural sources of fiber. Our Pritikin nutritionists stress BYOBB (no, they're *not* talking about alcohol):

- **B** is for beans (½ cup cooked = about 5 to 6 grams)
- **Y** is for yams (½ cup cooked = 3 to 5 grams)
- **O** is for oats (½ cup cooked = 3 to 5 grams)
- **B** is for barley (½ cup cooked = 3 to 5 grams)
- **B** is for berries (1 cup = about 5 grams)

A Word About "Superfoods"

People in America have gotten into a lot of trouble focusing on the latest "superfood," often generated by the media and million-dollar marketing budgets of the food industry. There's loads of money generated by shouting that Froot Loops with Strawberries have "more fiber," but little money for recommending that real fiber starts in the supermarket produce aisle.

The "superfoods" of this world are *not* soy nuts or dark chocolate or pomegranate juice; foods like these get 15 minutes of fame. Fruits, veggies, beans, and whole grains have had thousands of years of fame. They're the true superfoods.

KEY POINTS TO REMEMBER

- Start your meals with a super salad or soup or both.
- Whenever you can, replace your lunch or dinner with a giant salad filled with greens, colorful vegetables, beans, and/or lean protein such as white-meat poultry or tuna.
- All vegetables and fruits are good choices, but as a general rule of thumb, choose the darker varieties, which pack more nutrients.
- End your meals with fruit rather than dessert.
- Choose fresh, whole fruit instead of juice or dried fruit.
- Aim to consume at least 30 grams of fiber daily.

6

Pritikin Essential Ingredient 2: Eliminate High-Calorie Beverages

WE LIVE IN a culture of grande lattes, sports drinks, exotic-sounding bottled juices, and sweetened fruit "teas." Fancy coffee chains abound, as do refrigerator cases stocked with icy soft drinks; nearly everywhere you turn, you see people walking or driving with one of these beverages in hand. We rate cars by the number of cup holders, which now come heated and cooled. Without question, we're a nation of high-calorie beverage guzzlers, and though these drinks may taste good, we're paying a hidden cost.

One in every five calories in our American diet comes from beverages. When we were a thinner country, "beverages" meant water, tea, and coffee. Frozen blended drinks had not been invented yet. Based on scientific observation alone, soft drinks are guilty of contributing to the fattening of America. Soft-drink consumption has increased almost threefold in the past 20 years. Can you guess what else has radically increased over the past two decades? That's right: the size of our derrières.

As always, the proof is in the scientific research. A recent study of 91,000 nurses compared weight changes between drinkers of regular and diet drinks. After eight years, the regular beverage drinkers weighed 17 pounds more, as compared to the diet drinkers, who on average weighed only two pounds more. The nurses who switched to diet beverages halfway through the study nearly stopped gaining weight. Another study, of Massachusetts schoolchildren, showed that one additional soft drink per day increased the risk of obesity by 60 percent.

What explains the association between caloric soft drinks and obesity? First, research has shown that calories consumed in beverages provide far less satiety than the same amount of calories from solid foods. Calories in beverages are less filling, so you end up consuming more calories on days when they are consumed in drinks. In addition, most soft drinks contain high-fructose corn syrup, which is 30 percent sweeter than sucrose, or cane sugar. The simple truth is that most people like sweet foods and beverages. As you already know, high-fructose corn syrup doesn't induce leptin, a key hormone that signals us to eat less. According to our satiety detectors, it's like that drink never happened. According to our waistlines, though, there's no question of doubt.

Soft drinks, whether made with sugar or high-fructose corn syrup, are liquid calories. And liquid calories are a big problem if you're trying to lose weight because they are less satiating or filling, and so we don't compensate for them by eating less food later in the day. Indeed, while fruit juices are certainly better nutritionally than soft drinks, most contain about the same amount of sugar as soft drinks and are probably just as fattening. If you want to feel full on fewer calories, eat whole fruits and skip the juices.

In a fascinating study conducted by Purdue University in 2000, men and women were given 450 extra calories per day as either soft drinks or jelly beans, each for a month. Candy eaters ate less food to compensate for the extra calories, but soft-drinkers did not. Does this absolutely prove that caloric beverages are making us fat? No, not technically. But it does show that sugar-laden beverages are adding calories to our diets without signaling our hunger control mechanisms to compensate for those extra calories. And, as we already well know, weight gain is directly attributed to an excess of calories consumed.

CASE STUDY: KIRK

Kirk hadn't seen a doctor in years, although his Dunlap's Syndrome was obvious to everyone. This common malady is when the belly dun laps over the belt. He wore a size 42 belt but measured 46 inches around his waist. Kirk finally came to see me when he could no longer walk up a flight of stairs.

I had bad news for Kirk. He had all five features of metabolic syndrome: central obesity; high blood pressure, sugar, and triglycerides; and low HDL (good) cholesterol. His triglycerides of 4,000 were so high that a white layer rose to the top of his blood-sample tube like cream on raw milk. Although Kirk turned out not to have advanced coronary artery blockages, his heart had been weakened by years of uncontrolled high blood pressure. That's why he was so short of breath.

Kirk swore he ate very little, but on cross-examination admitted to drinking five or six 16-ounce bottles of regular cola each day. It never occurred to him that he was drinking in excess of 1,200 calories per day, or more than half the total calories he needed.

I convinced Kirk to switch to diet cola. Although he disliked it at first, after a few months he admitted that it wasn't so bad. Right now we're working on the next step, which is replacing some of the cola with water and coffee.

Kirk lost 20 pounds and two inches around the waist in three months without making any other changes. His triglycerides dropped to 400, which is not great, but certainly a lot better than 4,000! He needs only one instead of two medications to control his blood pressure, and he is much less short of breath.

SWITCHING TO WATER, DIET, AND SKIM

As evidenced by Kirk, cutting out calorie-laden beverages is one of the easiest ways to lose weight. On average, Americans drink almost 300 unnecessary and unhealthy calories each day, or 100,000 each year, in the form of sugar-dense soft drinks. If you currently drink at least two eight-ounce caloric beverages per day and switch to water, diet soda, or skim milk (in your coffee or by itself), you'll have found an easy way to cut out 200 calories per day. It's an easy calorie reduction that won't make you any hungrier.

We know your objections. First, you think that artificial sweeteners in diet drinks will kill you because they are not "natural." In fact, however, diet drinks are quite a bit safer than sugar-rich obesity- and diabetes-generating beverages. While some artificial sweeteners like saccharin have been loosely linked to cancer in male rats when given in extremely high doses, all the well-designed studies that have attempted to link artificial sweeteners to cancer in humans have found absolutely no association. Nor is there any data linking any artificial sweetener with headaches, nausea, stomach problems, or other symptom or disease. The Food and Drug Administration closely watches these widely used food additives and has concluded that there is no health risk. In contrast, being overweight or obese is likely to kill you. This is one clear instance where artificial beats natural—assuming you can call refined sugars "natural." On each dining-room table at the Pritikin Longevity Center are packets of noncaloric sweetener. We encourage you to dump out your sugar bowl at home and fill it with the little no-calorie packets instead.

Second, you don't like the taste of diet drinks. I encourage you, though, to try to change to an equivalent diet drink (diet soda for regular soda, or coffee with skim milk or soymilk and sweetener rather than cream and sugar) for two or three months. Like most of the guests we see at Pritikin who need to make this change, you might hate the taste for the first month but will tolerate it for the next month, and after two or three months, sugar-dense drinks will taste sickly sweet.

We can get used to almost anything we eat. Milk is a good example. The first time I tried skim milk, it tasted like water. After drinking skim milk for decades now, 1 percent fat milk tastes like cream to me. The same is true of diet drinks. Our tastes adapt in a few months; if you haven't given diet beverages a long enough trial, try again.

The Dangers of Soft Drinks for Children

Besides the obesity risks, soft drinks pose two threats for our youngsters:

1. Children often replace milk with soft drinks, reducing their calcium intake, and
2. Colas leach the calcium out of bones. One observational study found that bone fractures are five times as likely in girls who drink mostly colas rather than milk.

The good news is that we're making great strides in getting soft drinks out of our schools. The Clinton Foundation and the American Heart Association brokered a historic agreement with the major beverage producers just as this book neared publication. Beginning in fall 2008, beverages for sale in elementary and middle schools will be limited to milk, water, and juice with no sugar added. High schools will also have diet or low-calorie soft drinks and sports drinks. Students may still bring their own unhealthy beverages to school, and the issue of junk food has not yet been addressed. It's a real start, however, on fulfilling the second Pritikin lifestyle essential.

RATING BEVERAGES

Some of you may be surprised that we are not recommending going straight from regular soft drinks to water. Water would certainly be healthier, but few people can make that drastic a change right away. If you can, of course, switch directly to water, tea, and coffee. Skim or soymilk wouldn't hurt, either.

What are the best and worst beverages? Let's take a closer look at the facts.

Soft Drinks

At the top of the charts for worst beverages are, of course, sugar-packed soft drinks, because they contain a lot of calories and no nutrients.

Fruit Juice

Fruit juices are also loaded with sugar (in amounts similar to soft drinks, in fact); most "fruit drinks" are basically just sugar water plus some flavoring and a tiny amount of real fruit juice. But, unlike soft drinks, fruit juices at least contain some vitamins, minerals, and beneficial phytochemicals. Mixing juice with water reduces the caloric load and satisfies thirst better.

Sports Drinks

Sports drinks have about one-third less sugar than typical soft drinks, but they still are too high in salt and sugar. They vary considerably in added nutrients. Bottom line: Most sports drinks are still loaded with calories and salt—two things most Americans need to consume less of. Other than skim milk, soymilk, and alcohol (in moderation), it's never a good idea to drink calories, regardless of the source.

Coffee

Caffeinated coffee reduces hunger a bit, which assists weight loss to a very small measure. Excess caffeine, however, causes fast heart rhythms and raises blood pressure. A few studies have found more heart disease in people who drink more than five cups of coffee per day, but that appears to be due to substances in coffee (diterpenes) that increase LDL cholesterol levels in the blood. A paper filter removes most of these diterpenes and appears to lessen or eliminate the modest increased risk of heart disease. Moderate coffee drinking probably has little effect on heart disease provided it has passed through a paper filter and is consumed without cream or sugar.

Tea

Tea has less caffeine than coffee, and also contains several potentially beneficial antioxidants. Asian tea-drinking countries, such as Japan, typically have less heart disease. European tea-drinking countries, such as the United Kingdom, have a lot of heart disease, but they add milk to their tea. (As a general rule, it's best to never eat like the British.) Caseins in milk block the absorption of beneficial phytochemicals in tea and undo some of their anti-inflammatory benefits.

In the United States, moderate tea drinkers who suffer from heart attacks die 28 percent less often than non–tea drinkers; heavy tea drinkers die 44 percent less often. A possible explanation for the reduced heart disease is that tea increases nitric oxide release from the endothelium (blood cell walls). Our laboratory has shown that green tea has a slightly more beneficial effect on the endothelium than black tea, but both work and are great beverages.

Alcohol

Alcoholic beverages have complex health effects. Alcohol hampers weight loss because it adds calories and stimulates hunger. It has more calories per ounce than sugar. Drinking less alcohol is often the only change some heavy drinkers need to lose weight.

On the other hand, modest alcohol consumption (seven drinks per week for men and four per week for women) is good for your heart, even if it is not good for your waistline. Alcohol increases HDL (good) cholesterol about as effectively as exercise (no, this does not mean you can trade your treadmill for a case of merlot). Heavy drinking (more than 20 drinks per week), however, increases blood pressure and triglycerides, and in some cases weakens heart muscle.

Best and Worst Beverages for Weight Loss

Best: water, flavored water, sugar-free tea and coffee, skim milk, soymilk

OK: diluted fruit juice and sugar-free soft drinks

Worst: sugar-dense soft drinks, juice drinks with sugar added, 1%, 2%, and whole milk, alcohol (in excess of 1 drink per day)

KEY POINTS TO REMEMBER

- Sugar-dense soft drinks are making us fat, because they add calories without making us feel any fuller.
- Reducing your soft-drink intake by 16 ounces per day eliminates more than 200 unnecessary nutrient-free calories daily.
- Water, tea, skim milk, soymilk, and coffee (with noncaloric sweetener and skim milk or soymilk only) are the best beverage choices.
- Fruit juices are just as high in sugar and probably as fattening as soft drinks. Stick to whole fruits instead.
- Alcohol should be consumed only modestly

7

Pritikin Essential Ingredient 3: Trim Portions of Calorie-Dense Foods

NOW THAT YOU are eating more good-quality salads and soups, you'll have no trouble cutting down on calorie-dense food. The key concept here is that you want to reduce lunch and dinner by about 100 calories each: not by counting those calories, but by following Pritikin essential #1: *filling up on calorie-light, nutrient-dense foods first so you naturally have less appetite for the heavier stuff.* Then, you're able to practice portion control more easily.

PORTION CONTROL

This third lifestyle essential requires some fine-tuning (okay, complete revision) of our understanding of food portions. Americans now eat ridiculously large servings of food, many times the suggested portion. Potatoes are a good example, since they are America's favorite vegetable. On average, we eat our own weight in potatoes every year, or about 150 pounds. More than 50 pounds per person are gobbled up in one of the worst forms, French fries. Nutritionists define one portion of fries as 10 slices, or about 130 calories. Yet a "small" order of fries from a typical fast-food restaurant has grown to about one and a half standard portions, or 205 calories. A "large" order is about four to five times the standard portion size, or about 610 calories.

Just to put two "large" fast-food portions into perspective: two large orders of fries and two 16-ounce regular soft drinks provide enough calories to sustain a 135-pound person for an entire day without eating anything else. Of course, no one exists on just two orders of fries and two soft drinks in a typical day, which is exactly why 135-pound Americans are an endangered species.

Portion size in our country is clearly out of control. I recently picked up a small bag of American-made corn chips, obviously meant for one person. Its food label read 160 calories, which most people would assume was the number of calories in the package. Problem is, the bag contained 2.5 portions, so the actual number of calories is 400. In terms of calories that's more than a "snack"; that's almost a meal.

A comparison of restaurant portions around the world documents that American portions are ubiquitously super-sized. One recent trial compared portion sizes in Philadelphia and Paris. Compared to Parisian restaurants, Philadelphian restaurants served 25 percent larger average food portions and 52 percent larger soft drinks. Parisians also spent 55 percent more time eating and enjoying their smaller meals.

The last time I was in Philadelphia, I ate dinner in an excellent restaurant specializing in prime rib. Their specialty was at least an inch thick and covered the entire plate. It weighed 32 ounces, excluding the mashed potatoes swimming in butter on the side. The meal would have been considered a rude joke anywhere else in the world. The last time I checked, gluttony was still number six out of seven on the all-time hit parade of deadly sins.

CASE STUDY: JOHN TIMOTHY GANNON

"I'm kind of an old-timer at Pritikin," laughs John Timothy Gannon, 59, founder of Outback Steakhouse, Inc. Tim is known as "The Chef" at Outback Steakhouse corporate headquarters in Tampa, Florida, where he heads up research and development for more than 1,200 Outback restaurants worldwide.

Tim first came to the Pritikin Longevity Center nearly 20 years ago. His first couple of days, he had a tough time climbing the five flights of stairs to his hotel room to check his phone messages. "I was panting by the second flight," he says. But at the end of two weeks, he recalls, "I was *running* up all five flights."

Over the last several years, Tim's cardiovascular system has been transformed, too. His cholesterol, which started at 289, is now down to 109! Atherosclerotic plaques in his coronary arteries have disappeared.

So what's it like to be a steak guy *and* a Pritikin guy? Life is all about balance, says Tim. "Sure, you can indulge yourself with a great steak dinner—*once in a while.* But you can't go out every night and have three glasses of wine, a glass of champagne, a bloomin' onion, and a porterhouse."

Tim has learned, as you will, that you can eat very well—and very close to the Pritikin guidelines—every night at many restaurants. "At Pritikin, I took a whole group to the Outback Steakhouse near the Center, and we had a great meal—totally Pritikin. Big green salads with tangy tomato (fat-free) dressing, grilled chicken breast, seared salmon, baked potatoes, sweet potatoes, fresh steamed vegetables, and a glass of wine.

"It's never about any one particular food," he explained. "It's about making dozens of good choices throughout your day: picking up an apple for a snack instead of potato chips, choosing water with lemon slices and a little Splenda instead of cola, ordering sorbet rather than ice cream. Hey, a great peach can make you feel just as wonderful—better!—than a bag of Cheetos."

HELPFUL SUGGESTIONS FOR
HEALTHY PORTIONS

If a former steak-and-potatoes guy like John Timothy Gannon can do it,
you can, too! Here are some of the tips we teach guests at Pritikin:

- Practice smart portion control by trimming portions of calorie-
dense foods before you start eating. Make the decision about how
much to eat of these fattening foods before you take the first bite.
Then, *get rid of the rest.* Especially when you eat out or take home
prepared food, put about a quarter to half of each calorie-dense
dish on a separate plate and discard it. You may have been taught
that throwing away food is a sin, but it keeps farmers in business
and you healthy.

- My wife taught me this next crucial step: after you remove a quarter to half of a calorie-dense dish, *make it immediately inedible.* If
it remains within your reach in edible form, you will eventually
eat it. My wife and I love gooey chocolate desserts. When we dine
out, we order one to share between the two of us. We each take
three or four bites and then pour pepper on the rest. After the
pepper, we won't eat any more dessert no matter how long we lin-
ger at the table.

- Don't let other people size your servings. Your mother may love
you, but she tried her best to make you fat. In mother-think, a
chubby kid is a job well done. The food industry measures its success the same way. You shouldn't. Make sure you are the one in
control of how much is on your plate.

- You have no excuse for taking excessively large helpings of calorie-
dense food in your own kitchen. Cook less of them. Serve them
on smaller plates and the portions will seem larger. I purposely
use a small cereal bowl in the morning so that the fruit on top is
almost falling off. When I use a larger bowl, I just fill it—and eat
more! My wife and I use teeny-weenie bowls for ice cream and it
feels like a treat.

- Serve food attractively. Smaller portions of well-presented foods taste and satisfy you better. The Japanese are masters at presenting small portions of foods beautifully. They are also a whole lot thinner than Americans. Prepared, TV-type dinners should be limited to barracks and prisons. Food arranged on a plastic plate in little compartments signals you have fallen into culinary hell.

- Never put your whole meal out on the table at once. Eat it in courses and, as you learned through essential 1, start with something filling and calorie-light like a salad or soup. In restaurants, go ahead and ask for a salad that's two or three times the size that the restaurant normally serves. Ideally, then, you're not feeling hungry at all by the time your calorie-dense entrée is served.

- As a parent, remember that serving large food portions is not a loving gesture. Love is bringing up slim, healthy, happy kids.

- Choose restaurants that serve smaller portions. Generally, smaller portions mean that the food is better in quality and better-tasting. Boycott restaurants that advertise all-you-can-eat unless 10 visits qualify you for free liposuction, stomach stapling, or bypass surgery.

- Buffets are coronary disasters and waistline killers. Grazing over acres of food almost guarantees overeating. Cruises often serve buffets and keep them open all hours of the night. I've often thought cruises should be rated by average weight gained, such as "Five Pounders," "Ten Pounders," and "Bury Me at Sea" extravaganzas.

- You can ask for half portions in restaurants, especially good ones. Or order one or two appetizers (soup and big salad, anyone?) instead of a large entrée.

- Share food. Most American restaurant entrées easily satisfy two people. A large order of fast-food fries—which, as we know, is not healthy or good for weight loss by any standard—serves four or five people. The entire table can share the average restaurant dessert. Besides, three extra spoons are a lot cheaper than three more desserts (or new pants in a bigger size).

- Take food home from restaurants. Retired people know fully well that this saves money. Give it to your dog, or eat it tomorrow. Recently, I shared a plate-overlapping, inch-thick prime rib from a famous restaurant with a 250-pound dog. Guess who got three-quarters?
- Send excess food back to the kitchen. Make a comment to your waiter. The chef may finally get the right idea.

KEY POINTS TO REMEMBER

- Trim your caloric intake at meals by first filling up on calorie-light foods, such as soups and salads.
- Avoid temptation by trimming your serving size of calorie-dense food before your first bite and then make the remainder inedible, immediately.
- Adjust your portion sizes of calorie-dense meals at home by preparing less food, using smaller serving plates, and arranging/presenting food attractively.
- Adjust your portion sizes of calorie-dense meals in restaurants by ordering less and/or cutting your portion in half, avoiding "all you can eat" scenarios, visiting higher-quality restaurants, and sharing your food with others. If necessary and appropriate, take home a doggie bag.
- Remember that heaping portions or a clean plate does not equal love. Show your love for those around you in other ways.

8

Pritikin Essential Ingredient 4: Snack Smarter

WE HAVE FOOD everywhere, and we eat it everywhere. Not only are we snacking more frequently, we are eating more calorie-dense snacks. The average snack has increased by 50 calories over the past 20 years, and our increased snacking of junk food is responsible for about 75 percent of the calories Americans have added to their diet during this period.

There are good reasons why we shouldn't graze all day on junk food. Almost any fatty or sugary food reduces nitric oxide, and refined carbohydrate-induced insulin resistance accelerates atherosclerosis. Most health evidence suggest that we should eat less frequently; we know from experiments that animals are more stress-resistant if they fast periodically. We also know that none of this scientific information is likely to make you stop snacking. Keep reading!

WHY WE SNACK

Snacking is driven by three simple factors:

1. Habit
2. Food availability
3. Eating low-satiety foods at meals

We've already tackled number three on this list in the first three Pritikin essentials; by now, you should be well on your way to enjoying calorie-light, nutrient-packed, beautifully presented foods at meals so that you feel full and satisfied. Now let's see what we can do about numbers one and two, which really go hand in hand.

A Matter of Habit

We eat out of habit almost as much as we eat to alleviate hunger. Certain activities trigger snack associations automatically in America: movies and buttered popcorn, ball games and Cracker Jacks or hot dogs, airline flights and peanuts or pretzels. For many people, snacking goes hand in hand with their everyday activities; they reach for the snacks almost without thinking—the late-morning donut, the three o'clock monster-size cookie, the handful of crackers or chips while watching evening television. Some people snack in the car, others while sitting at their desk, still others at recreational moments. One patient simply couldn't imagine enjoying her favorite spy novels every night without a handful of Twizzlers by her side, which she would chew through on autopilot.

CASE STUDY: MARK

Mark is a big boy. At 15 years old, he already weighed 250 pounds. Unlike most kids, Mark rarely ate fast food, but he did live in a house that had junk food everywhere—and I mean *everywhere.* The cabinets were stocked with every imaginable variety of cookie, "cheez" cracker, cream-filled "baked good," and salty, trans fat–laden snack food. Not surprisingly, Mark reacted to the open access to food like most of us do. He ate constantly.

Mark's mother eventually did two smart things: she removed most of the junk food in the house, replacing it with healthier alternatives, and told Mark that he couldn't get his driver's license until he lost 30 pounds. No problem! Some changes to the source of the problem and really good motivation solved Mark's weight issue in a few months. Mark finally got his license . . . and a few more female friends, as well.

Fighting Off Snack Attacks

Poor snacking habits are not necessarily easy to break, but like Mark, with a little motivation (weight loss and heart health) and understanding of the problem (too many snacks available too much of the time), you absolutely can do it.

Here are a few Pritikin hints that will help you resist reaching for sugary, salty, fattening snacks between meals.

- Start by getting rid of the junk food and snacks around the house, office, or car. If it isn't there, you won't be so tempted. Snacking is a habit and keyed response that can, over time and with diligence, be rewired.
- If you must have food within your reach 24/7, make it healthy food such as fruit and vegetables. Bowls of fruit within reach can be comforting to people trying to lose weight, even if they are never touched. To paraphrase Yogi Berra, dieting is "90 percent mental—the other half is physical." The Pritikin Center always has big bowls of ripe, colorful fruit around, day and night.
- Before leaving home every day, pack a few of the healthy, filling snacks you'll find a little later in this chapter so that you're "armed" when hunger hits. It will make all the difference to your weight-loss goals! For one thing, you'll be able to resist the temptation to pull into the fast-food drive-through lane for "a little something." A Burger King Whopper has 760 calories; a big, juicy, appetite-

satisfying apple that you can simply toss into your handbag or briefcase before you leave the house has just 100.

- Unless you are truly hungry, do something else when you get a food craving between meals. Focus your mind and energy elsewhere. For instance, take a break and call an emotionally nourishing friend or loved one at three p.m. instead of wolfing down a cookie. I used to come home from work and start grazing long before dinner was ready. Now I walk around my neighborhood or, in bad weather, watch the news while walking on the treadmill. As an added bonus, after walking, I'm less hungry when I sit down to eat dinner.
- If you know that you will want to snack later, postpone eating part of a reasonable meal until later. For instance, instead of eating cereal and yogurt for breakfast, eat the cereal and have the yogurt mid-morning.
- If you truly are hungry, have some veggies, fruit, or nonfat yogurt pre-meal. Eating a light, healthy snack has been shown to decrease total calorie intake.

MAKING GOOD SNACK CHOICES

Ask Dr. Bob

Question: Should I avoid snacking altogether between meals?

Answer: Not necessarily, as long as you are snacking smart. For most people, eating two or three reasonable meals per day with an occasional healthy snack is the best approach to staying satisfied and still losing weight.

The key, of course, is to make better snack choices, which is the main thing we teach guests at Pritikin. We have one main "don't" when it comes to choosing a snack: ditch the dry stuff. As much as you can, steer clear of dry snacks like potato chips, crackers, candy bars, trail mix, cookies, energy bars, and even healthier choices like bagels, pretzels, and fat-free baked chips. All dry foods pack a whole lot of calories into very small packages.

As for snacking "do's," there are many! Take a look below, and we think you'll quickly see that there is a whole wide world of better snack options out there.

Fresh fruit: If you're pressed for time, buy convenient, easy-to-wash, easy-to-peel varieties, such as tangerines, apples, bananas, grapes, and peaches. Even easier (though pricier) are pre-cut slices of fruit, such as watermelon and pineapple, in small plastic containers in the produce section of many supermarkets. Pick up your fresh fruit while picking up your greens and veggies at the supermarket salad bar.

Fresh veggies: Choose easy-to-prepare ones, like cherry tomatoes, red bell peppers, and celery. Buy pre-cleaned and cut veggies in the produce section, such as single-serving bags of baby carrots or celery (bring two or three bags with you) or use a container from your supermarket's salad buffet. Keep balsamic vinegar or another favorite Pritikin dressing in the office refrigerator for quick salad snacks.

Hearty bean-rich soups: Great choices include black bean, minestrone, and lentil soups. Make your own (see recipes in Part Three) and freeze in easy-to-carry single-serving containers, or buy them frozen from the pritikin.com store. Soups with a small amount of meat, fish, or poultry are also great for curbing your appetite and shedding weight. At the office, just pop your soup in the microwave. Alternatively, pack store-bought low-sodium varieties, such as cans of Pritikin or Healthy Valley, or Tabatchnick, located in the frozen-food section of markets.

Yogurt: Look for nonfat, no sugar/syrup varieties, such as Dannon Light & Fit, Stonyfield Farm (plain), and fat-free, plain Greek-style yogurts like Oikos and Fage. Sweeten plain varieties naturally with fresh, cut-up fruit, such as strawberries and bananas.

Baked potatoes: Many markets now have baked (russet) potatoes individually shrink-wrapped and prewashed. All you do is microwave one for 7 or 8 minutes. Healthy, calorie-light toppings include fat-free sour cream, mustard, red pepper flakes, and low-sodium salsa (such as Enrico's, Garden Valley, or Trader Joe's varieties). Even better, throw some broccoli in with the salsa or sour cream.

Sweet potato "fries": Look in the refrigerated sections of markets such as Trader Joe's and big-box stores such as Costco for bags of fresh sweet potatoes prewashed and cut in the shape of French fries. They are also available from Mann Packing Company in California (www.veggies madeeasy.com). Just throw some on a nonstick cookie sheet, sprinkle with a little garlic powder and black pepper, and bake.

Corn on the cob: Microwave, husk and all, for 3 to 5 minutes.

Corn tortillas: Warm one or two tortillas between slightly moistened towels in a microwave, then top with lettuce, diced onions, a little salsa, and bean dip, and fold. Tasty low-sodium bean-dip brands include Bearitos and Guiltless Gourmet.

Oatmeal: Oatmeal or another hot cereal for an afternoon snack? Why not? All you need is the oatmeal (no-salt-added brands include Bob's Red Mill and Arrowhead Mills), water, and a bowl. If you'd like, add a little nonfat milk and sliced banana. As the saying goes, it'll "stick to your ribs" till dinner.

Pop-top canned fruits: Buy the varieties packed in juice or water, no sugar added. Good brands include Del Monte and Dole.

Frozen snacks/meals: Great ready-in-minutes choices include veggie burgers like Gardenburger Garden Vegan (lower in sodium than other brands), Hash Browns (Cascadian Farms or Simply Potatoes), and Roasted Vegetable Pizza (Advantage/10).

The chefs at the Pritikin Longevity Center prepare and send frozen meals worldwide to Pritikin alumni and friends. They're the same soups, entrées, snacks, and desserts prepared and served at Pritikin. For more information, call 800-327-4914 or visit the store at pritikin.com.

If you have a minute or two to prepare a tasty, satisfying snack, try the following combinations:

Baked potato and chili: Just pour vegetarian chili or your favorite soup over your baked potato for a quick, hearty meal or snack. (A good brand of canned vegetarian chili is Health Valley.)

Corn and salsa: Simply microwave frozen no-salt-added corn and mix in fresh salsa. Make it even more fiber-rich and heartier by adding canned low-sodium beans and diced red peppers.

Tuna and whole-grain crackers: Combine canned tuna and fresh pre-washed baby spinach. Spoon over a couple of Kavli or Wasa Crispbreads. The only effort involved is opening the can of tuna.

Soup and veggies: Thicken and flavor your soup by adding veggies. For example, add to a big bowl of lentil soup a box of microwaved frozen spinach. Easy!

Yogurt and fruit: Stir fresh sliced bananas and strawberries into nonfat plain yogurt. Easier yet, open a can of no-sugar-added fruit such as Del Monte and mix with your yogurt.

Beans and just about anything: Keep a ready supply of no-salt-added canned beans such as pinto and cannellini beans. Pour over salads, tortillas, pastas, baked potatoes, rice, soups, you name it.

Pitas and just about anything: Stuff a whole-wheat pita (good low-sodium brands are Toufayan Bakeries and Garden of Eatin' Pitettes) or top low-sodium whole-wheat bread with just about anything already in the fridge or pantry, such as fresh cucumber and other veggies, hummus, fresh turkey breast (oven-roasted, deli-style, no salt), salmon (canned, rinsed, unsalted), or fat-free cheese. Good fat-free cheese brands include Alpine Lace, Lifetime, and Smart Bea. Use the cheeses sparingly, because they're fairly high in sodium.

Lastly, if you have a little more time to prepare delicious snacks, you'll find several tasty recipes in the "Snacks, Salads, and Side Dishes" section of Part Three.

Happy snacking!

KEY POINTS TO REMEMBER

- Snacking on junk food is making you fat. Period.
- Mindless snacking is a habit that can be broken. Snack smarter!
- Clear out the junk food; if it isn't there, you won't eat it.
- It's not *whether* you snack, but *what* you snack on that matters.
- Ditch the dry stuff; packaged snack foods like pretzels, chips, and cookies—even the "low-fat" varieties—pack a lot of calories.
- Keep delicious healthy snacks on hand so you aren't tempted by the junk.

9

Pritikin Essential Ingredient 5: Forget Fast Food; Dine Unrefined

IN A PERFECT world, we would gather fresh fruits, vegetables, nuts, and whole grains, cook them if necessary, and eat them. If we were lucky, we would catch a fish or bird, cook it, and add it to the meal. Unfortunately, the last time we could actually live like that year-round was in the Garden of Eden. After that came winter, drought, pests, cities, periodic hunger and famine, and the Industrial Revolution. Preserving food was one of man's greatest achievements ... almost. Sure, refrigeration and canning are wonderful. But trans fat–laden doughnuts, which can remain fresh on a shelf for months, end up shortening *your* shelf life.

Don't get me wrong; I like my milk skimmed, pasteurized, and vitamin D enriched. I have no argument with adding folic acid to cereals and breads to reduce birth defects. I'm certainly not against all food processing and preservation. But what started as a means of survival and convenience has turned to deadly excess. Whole grains have been stripped naked of nutrients. The salt, sugar, and fat added to almost all processed foods for "taste" translates into a world of illness.

WHOLE VERSUS REFINED FOODS

Whole food refers to plant and animal food in its original form. At the complete opposite end of the spectrum is processed and refined food. Whole foods contain their full complement of vitamins, minerals, complex carbohydrates, fiber, and antioxidants, many of which are lost in processing. Food processing may help preserve foods, but it can also remove nutrients and fiber. Preservation of food isn't all bad: preserving by heating is generally okay; preserving with salt or fat hydrogenation is not.

Processed Produce

I am quite sure that if the Garden of Eden were created today, Eve would be tempted with a French fry or potato chip, not an apple. Food processing has gone way beyond simple food preservation. Routinely add fat, sugar, and salt to a perfectly acceptable potato and before long you have obesity, diabetes, and high blood pressure. Need some ketchup on your fries? The added salt and sugar have destroyed a perfectly good tomato. Fully 90 percent of the calories from ketchup come from refined sugar. (If you want a healthier ketchup, go to Pritikin's store at www.pritikin.com: the Pritikin ketchup is low in salt and sugar, and made of *real* tomatoes!)

Try to get to know the produce section of your supermarket. There you'll find the original Garden of Eden, full of fresh potatoes, tomatoes, greens, and so on before the salt, sugar, bacon bits, and gobs of dressing smothered them.

Refined Grains

Refining grains is almost never a good idea. Wheat, rice, oats, cornmeal, and barley start as whole grains containing bran, germ, and endosperm. Most of the vitamins, minerals, and other micronutrients are contained in the bran and germ. Refining grains strips off the bran and germ, leaving the starchy endosperm. This produces a finer texture—hence the term "refined"—but reduces nutrients. White flour and white rice are examples of refined grains. Many refined grains are enriched with a few vitamins, but they never have the original complete nutritional package. "Enriched" grains can never equal the nutritional value of unrefined whole grains.

How do you know which products on the market are whole and which are refined? By reading the packaging. The first ingredient should have the word *whole* right there in it: whole grain, whole wheat, etc. (or it should say "brown rice"). *Multigrain, organic, enriched, degerminated, durum,* or *semolina* does not mean whole grain. Make sure that the *first* grain listed is a whole grain; if the second grain listed is "whole," the product may contain almost no whole grain.

FAST FOOD

At the most deadly end of the food spectrum is fast food. Is fast food really bad for us? The answer to this question is about as definitive as knowing that the Pope is Catholic. Here are a few illustrative facts:

- The average fast-food meal contains 1,050 calories. Fast-food portions only vary from too large to ridiculously too large.
- Fat and sugar make up three-quarters of fast-food calories. The average fast-food meal contains 41 grams of fat, much of it saturated. Saturated fat is the major cause of high total cholesterol and high LDL (bad) cholesterol in our society.
- Fast-food chains typically fry their food in killer oils. A very pop-

ular chain's large order of French fries currently contains eight grams of trans fat. That's more in one dish than you should eat in a week.

- Heart-healthy whole grains, fruits, and vegetables are endangered menu items in fast-food establishments.

- Fast food is, well, fast. You're done before you have any sense of what you've eaten, and long before you've given your stomach a chance to register that you're full (which you likely were halfway through).

- Fast food drive-ups are the ultimate form of physical inactivity. They are the adult equivalent of being nursed as a baby. For the record, valet parking is not much better.

- Data from our laboratory demonstrate that a typical fast-food meal injures an artery's lining, or endothelium, much like cigarette smoking does.

- White blood cell counts go up about 60 percent (hence inflammation) within two hours of eating a high-fat fast-food meal, about the same as with appendicitis. Remember, atherosclerosis is an inflammatory disease.

- In a recent study of young people, just walking into a fast-food restaurant twice or more per week resulted in a 10-pound weight gain after 15 years compared with those who rarely ate fast food.

- In the same study, fast-food frequenters were also twice as likely to become diabetic.

CASE STUDY: SAM

Sam is a drug salesman, in and out of doctors' offices all day long. Most of his breakfasts used to be egg sandwiches (often ones that came in Styrofoam boxes at the drive-thru), and his lunches cheeseburgers and fries. He frequently ate in his car. Sam played football in high school and was always a big man, six foot two and at least 250 pounds. But he knew his increasing weight was getting to be an issue.

After seeing the movie *Super-size Me*, Sam asked me whether fast food was part of his problem. I knew that he already knew the answer.

We laid out a new eating plan for Sam: hot cereal with fruit for break-fast—*at home*—and deli-bought small sandwiches and ready-made salads for lunch. I also asked him to park as far away as possible from the door of the offices he visited. Sam lost 34 pounds in the first six months of this plan and was still losing weight the last time I saw him. He credits the movie for chang-ing his life.

Better "Fast" Food Choices

When it comes to preparing healthy food, cooking at home is the best option, but if you don't have the time, what is the almost-as-fast, health-iest alternative to fast food? Just as Sam did, buy prepared food in a su-permarket or deli. It is not necessarily more expensive. I recently bought a tasty, whole skinned roasted chicken that would feed four people from an upscale "natural" grocery for less than $8. (It's not as healthy as cook-ing your own chicken breasts, because these chickens are usually loaded with salt, plus they have dark meat but they're certainly a better choice than KFC. Sorry, Colonel.) Add a prepared large salad, vegetables, and calorie-light beverage and you have a fairly healthy dinner for four peo-ple for less than $20.

Our Fast-Food Society

Our fast-food lifestyle is bad for us beyond the consequences of the food. In America, we eat for survival while we should dine for enjoy-ment. In less obese societies, people eat meals more slowly. You already know why, biologically, this is a good practice. The best way to eat slowly is to make meals social occasions, which also makes it a good emotional practice. Around the world, eating is the time that family, friends, and colleagues get together. We have lost the social enjoyment of eating. We eat while watching television, a habit that hardly encourages social in-teraction. Really take your time to taste the food and enjoy the companionship. If you do eat alone, don't watch TV. Read a newspaper or book, or just enjoy some quality quiet time.

Take the "fast food" approach out of your life, all the way around. Instead of racing from one thing to another, plan more enjoyable experiences. Go to an upbeat movie, play, concert, or sports event with a friend or family member. Work less, but more effectively. Romance your significant other more. Enjoy more intimate and sexual relations. People who regularly experience more enjoyable events in their lives weigh less. More importantly, their entire existence is happier. One of the greatest tragedies of our American lifestyle is that we have traded in happy lives for too-full stomachs. Sadly, what we're filling them with is not even very tasty food.

Attention, Parents!

You need to become role models for good lifestyle practices and appropriate weight for your children. If they see you frequently dining at the drive-through, guess where they are likely to head for lunch the instant they are of driving age? Know that every time you offer them fast food as a reward, you're creating second-generation fast-food junkies. If they start seeing you make better, healthier food choices, they will, too.

CASE STUDY: VALERIE AND FAMILY

Valerie, a family doctor, was working 10-hour days. At the end of those days, she didn't have much energy for her children, ages five and seven, and husband. Dinner was usually fast-food burgers or delivery pizza. Valerie was only 37, but she felt much older. She was on cholesterol medications, was carrying 30 extra pounds, and wasn't exercising. Her kids, to her horror, were getting plump, too. Her father, also a doctor, was a huge fan of the Pritikin Program, through which he'd lost more than 60 pounds. When Valerie decided to change her life, she took Dad's lead.

That was five years ago. Today Valerie is 128 pounds, size 6, and medication free. Her family life has changed, too. "We're having a lot of fun!" laughs Valerie. They've traded greasy pizzas for "build-your-own-burrito" nights where bowls of salsa, chicken breast strips, lettuce, and pinto beans get spread out on the kitchen table and family members create their own Mexican sensation.

Family time is now often synonymous with exercise time. Evenings and weekends, the whole gang is out in the front yard, shooting hoops. On the few evenings they watch TV, they take turns walking on the treadmill that's set up *in front* of the TV.

"Living Pritikin-style has given me that wonderful sense of feeling good, of *wanting* to get up each morning," says Valerie. "And now in the evenings I have plenty of energy to enjoy my family. That's a huge benefit."

KEY POINTS TO REMEMBER

- Always choose "whole" foods over refined foods: whole fruits and vegetables in their unprocessed form and unrefined grains.
- Any grain product you buy should have the word *whole* listed as the first ingredient.
- When approaching a drive-thru, drive right on past. Your health—and the health of your family—depends on it. Fast food is the deadliest form of refined, processed food there is.
- Delicious prepared foods are available at the deli counter of your local supermarket. While not as good for you as home-cooked food, they are a relatively inexpensive and quick alternative to fast food.

10

Pritikin Essential Ingredient 6: Watch Less, Walk More

WE LIVE IN a sedentary society, in which the size of our waistlines is increasing right along with the size of our big-screen televisions. In response, Pritikin essential #6 has a very simple message: *Put down the remote control and get moving!*

At the Pritikin Longevity Center, we do have televisions in each room, though we're consistently told by guests that by the end of their action-packed days here, they don't even bother turning them on. They are ready for bed! Virtually their entire day is spent doing some sort of physical activity. After breakfast, they're off to the exercise facilities for 45 minutes of cardio workouts on treadmills, exercycles, and other aerobic equipment, all supervised by Pritikin's university-degreed exercise physiologists. In various aerobic classes, guests whoop and holler to music with a beat (everything from Donna Summer to Red Hot Chili Peppers). Or maybe they head off to weight-lifting class, which is based on a very simple, 10-exercise format that can be performed just about anywhere, from home to hotel rooms (see Appendix A), then perhaps to yoga for "60 minutes of bliss," as many report. It's so blissful, in fact, that many end up fast asleep by the end of class, tucked under their yoga blankets. Between all this and other elective classes like Pilates, cardio-boxing, and salsa dancing, who has time for television?

As you've heard us say several times by this point, changing your lifestyle *on all levels* is necessary to lose weight and achieve true heart health. Remember, what you eat absolutely matters, but your level of physical activity is of equal importance. So turn off that TV set and get going!

CASE STUDY: TED

Ted lives in a very nice house surrounded by two acres of lawn. Every weekend, he would ride around on his mower, carrying a beer in hand. Can't you just picture him, earphones playing, smile on his face? This was his kingly domain.

Every year, Ted's lawn looked spectacular, but he managed to gain 10 pounds. Does this sound familiar? By age 50, he was carrying 240 pounds on his five-foot-ten frame, and his cholesterol exceeded his weight.

With considerable nudging from his good-looking wife and a little from me, Ted decided to lose weight. He dismounted his riding mower, parked it permanently in the garage, and bought a power walk-behind model. Ted now spends about an hour walking behind his mower four or five times a week. He doesn't have a free hand for a can of beer, but his earphones are still singing. He now weighs a little less than 200 pounds, and his cholesterol is about the same. Oh . . . and his lawn still looks spectacular.

THE EFFECTS OF EXERCISE

How much would you pay for a medication that made you happier and healthier, look better, and live longer? Probably a lot. What if we told you that physical activity would cost you a lot less—and was guaranteed to produce the same results? Our guess is that you'd quickly get rid of whatever your version of Ted's riding mower is and get moving.

We were meant to chase lunch, not order it. The only cause of heart disease that exercise doesn't improve is the bad genes you inherited from your parents. Briefly, physical activity:

- increases HDL (good) cholesterol
- reduces blood pressure
- reduces blood sugar
- reduces diabetes
- increases nitric oxide
- reduces inflammation and blood clotting
- retards atherosclerosis progression
- reduces heart attacks (and the mortality rate following a heart attack)
- reduces strokes
- reduces senility
- increases metabolic rate
- decreases appetite and food cravings
- burns calories
- reduces constipation
- reduces bone fractures
- improves appearance
- increases muscle mass
- increases sense of well-being
- decreases stress
- reduces depression
- increases mental sharpness
- increases longevity

Attention, Couch Potatoes!

How bad is being a couch potato? Well, the Nurses' Health Study evaluated daily activities over a six-year period and observed the following:

- Each hour per day of sedentary TV watching increased obesity by 12 percent.
- Each hour per day of sedentary work (i.e. sitting at a desk) increased obesity by 3 percent.
- Each hour per day of brisk walking reduced obesity by 14 percent.

Physical Activity and Heart Disease

One of the earliest studies to realize the cardiovascular benefit of physical activity took place on London's buses back in 1966. Fare-takers, constantly moving around the double-decker buses to collect money, had 30 percent fewer heart attacks than the seated drivers.

Another well-known study, the Honolulu Heart study, was the first to discover that the benefit of physical activity actually increases with age. That study found that elderly men who walked at least one and a half miles per day had 50 percent fewer heart attacks than those who did little walking. In comparison, middle-aged men had 17 percent fewer heart attacks. So you see, it's never too late!

Physical activity has a myriad of benefits in the fight against heart disease. It has a positive impact on nearly all the coronary risk factors, including reducing obesity, blood sugar, blood pressure, and inflammation, and increasing nitric oxide, and improving your overall emotional sense of well-being. As I said earlier, a pair of sneakers and a pedometer cost less than bypass surgery. Yes, perhaps I'm putting myself out of business as a cardiologist by encouraging this, but I'd far rather play golf any day than watch heart disease ruin lives.

Physical Activity and Longevity

The more active you are, the longer you'll live. It's that simple. The Harvard Alumni Study found that you live about a minute longer for every minute that you exercise. If you think this doesn't matter to you now, at this stage of your life, imagine how much all those extra minutes will mean when you're 80 and awaiting the birth of your great-grandchildren.

THOSE FEET WERE MADE FOR WALKING

Physical activity comes in two forms: lifestyle activities and exercise. Lifestyle activities, such as walking, house and yard chores, and manual work, used to be enough to keep people fit and trim. That is no longer true. Why? Because we ride lawn mowers, open garage doors with a click of a button, and wash our clothes and dishes in automated machines. We drive an average of 22 miles per day and park as close to where we are going as possible—that is, if we park at all, given our drive-thru restaurants, banks, churches, and coffee chains.

You have two choices: increase your lifestyle activities or start exercising. Ideally, we'd like to see you do both, but chances are you'll have a better chance of sticking with more lifestyle activities. Walking is the meat and potatoes of lifestyle activity. Your heart may be a little happier if you do some jogging, but your waistline doesn't much care whether you walk, jog, or crawl the same distance.

I know you think you walk a lot, but you probably don't. Spend $20 on your future and buy a pedometer. Using a pedometer gives you feedback, which is essential for any lifestyle change. I have one that talks to me. Every 1,000 steps, it announces how far I've walked that day. After you have purchased a pedometer, take a few days to determine how much you actually walk. I think you'll be surprised at how few steps you actually take each day.

Pedometers have proven value in getting people to walk more. It's hard to lie to the pedometer (although I've heard of a few people who shake theirs on the way home to register more steps). Ideally, you want to be logging 10,000 steps each day. Isn't 10,000 steps a lot of walking? Yes, it is about five miles. It takes about 90 minutes at a good pace if you walk it all at once, but since few of us have 90 minutes straight to devote to exercising, you can space it throughout your day.

Ask Dr. Bob

Question: How much do I need to walk each day to lose weight?

Answer: For the purposes of weight loss, I want you to add 3,500 to 4,000 steps to whatever you are currently walking every day, or about two miles. Walking even more steps per day would be better, but this 30 to 40 minutes' effort burns the necessary 200 additional calories to lose 20 pounds in a year.

Increasing the amount you walk each day starts by making an attitude shift. Walking can be one of the great enjoyments in life. Look around the cities of Europe and the busy, cosmopolitan cities in the United States such as New York, Chicago, and San Francisco. People of all ages are walking everywhere. Some are natives, happily talking to a coworker on their way to lunch or glancing into store windows; some are visitors, taking in the amazing sights. All around them are interesting scenery, smells, and people, all of which they would miss if they were behind the wheel of a car, battling traffic. When we walk, we are engaged with the world around us, whether it is city life or the sounds and smells in nature. We actually feel physically and emotionally better. We feel less stressed. We sleep better. We're just overall happier people when we're walking more, period.

A key component to increasing the amount you walk is viewing everyday activities in a different light—each one as a separate opportunity to log a few more steps. Though we touched on this in Chapter 2, it is such an essential part of our program that it bears repeating. Here are just some of the ways to incorporate more walking into your regular daily life:

- Purposely park as far away from the door as possible. I know that you are going to park in your garage or in front of your house, but all other times, use driving as an opportunity to walk. I'll bet the only time that you parked in the back of the lot was the day you bought your car. You didn't want it dinged. The next day you again parked right by the door. Look at the parking lots of athletic clubs. Even there, everyone parks as close to the entrance as possible. Then, as good Americans, they run on treadmills.

- Do not drive short distances. Walk. In this country, we drive any distance more than two or three blocks, at most. Walk to a store five blocks away and take a cart or backpack if you need to bring back something heavy. If your young children live within a mile of school, walk with them. Get them and you in the habit of walking. You golfers, walk the whole course, or at least park on the cart path and walk to your ball. That way you will get in some walking and find that you are less nervous standing over your shot. Golf, like life, was meant to be walked.

- Walk as a family. Walk to a park. Just walk around your neighborhood. Walking around your neighborhood is a great way to meet people and to stay in tune with your community and the seasons. Around the world, families actually go out for walks as enjoyment. In this country, if you saw a family of four walking along a road on a Sunday afternoon, you would probably call the police. Obviously, their car broke down. Otherwise, why would they be walking? Maybe they just want to be slim and healthy!

- Use stairs. Stairs are notched inclined surfaces for walking up and down. Some people use them so infrequently that I just thought I would remind you of their existence. Start by walking down and work up to routinely climbing three or four flights. Do not place objects at the bottom of a stairwell to take up on future trips; use the opportunity to walk the flight of stairs *now*. My mother did that until she was 95. Use it or lose it! One of my 70-year-old physician colleagues starts teaching rounds by walking from our third floor to our thirteenth floor. It takes the medical students with him about 10 minutes to catch their breath. You can bet that he asks them a whole bunch of questions while they are huffing and puffing. Increase your lifestyle activities while you are young and stick with them. A friend of mine knows a lady who climbs 15 floors to her apartment. She has to pass Condi Rice's Secret Service people every time and was always searched until they got used to her. She is 73 years old. What's your excuse?

- If you work in an office, get up from your chair every hour or so and walk somewhere. Carry a message instead of e-mailing it. Talk to someone. You might find that talking directly to coworkers gets more accomplished. People who are always moving about are called fidgety. Good studies demonstrate that fidgety people, who do a lot of lifestyle activity, are as protected from heart disease as are people who exercise regularly.

- Walk as briskly as possible. People who walk quickly have a lower risk of stroke and heart attack. The benefit of walking is most evident if you walk at least three miles per hour. Four miles per hour is even better. You do not need to walk a great distance at once. Three 10-minute walks are as good as one 30-minute walk. Incorporate more walking into your routine lifestyle, even if you're very busy. One of our Pritikin guests, U.S. Congressman Charles Rangel of New York, certainly has a lot on his plate, especially now as senior member of the Ways and Means Committee. Still, he often walks from the Capitol to his office instead of taking the subway. At least four times weekly, he climbs the 16 flights of stairs to his home. At 70-plus years, he still looks great! Congratulations, Charley!

- Do not use bad weather as an excuse not to walk. Go to a shopping mall and walk. Many shopping malls have walking clubs. They offer social opportunities and the group reinforces your commitment, or at least makes you feel guilty when you don't honor it. Just remember to leave your credit cards at home. When I'm staying at a hotel without an exercise room in a neighborhood I don't know, I simply walk the halls and stairs for 30 minutes. No matter how difficult the day, it makes me feel better.

- Another alternative to walking outside or in malls is using a treadmill. Treadmills are fine for very busy people. They are an excellent means for getting in the 10,000 steps, though they don't provide the enjoyment of scenery, seasons, and company.

Tips for Safe, Healthy Walking

In addition to the suggestions above, here are a few tips from our excellent exercise physiologists for those times when you are walking for exercise:

- Do not stretch before you walk. Walk a little to warm up your muscles, then stretch.
- Be sure to walk safely. That means away from traffic and dangerous areas. Always wear reflective or light-colored clothing at night. Ask people and/or walk with someone if you don't know whether the area is safe.
- Walk during the cool part of summer days and the warm part of winter days. Remember to bring along some water or stop for a drink.
- Wear comfortable shoes or sneakers and layered clothing. Just walking warms you up quite a bit, so wear top layers that are easy to remove.
- You generally do not need to consult your physician before walking more unless you already have heart disease. Your body will tell you when you are overdoing it. Chest pain, shortness of breath, dizziness, or cramps in the calf muscles during walking are symptoms that need medical attention. Expect some stiffness the day after you walk if you currently walk very little.

- Purposely walk more when you travel a long distance by car or airplane. Protracted sitting can cause blood clots in your legs. These blood clots can break free, travel to your lung, and kill you. Every hour or at most two while driving, get out of your car and walk. You will even stay more alert. While flying, get out of your seat periodically and walk up and down the aisle. That's what Nathan Pritikin, founder of the Pritikin Program, always did. He just smiled graciously if flight attendants gave him dirty looks for getting in the way of their beverage carts. (As an aside: consider taking an aspirin before a long car, plane, or train trip to reduce the chance of developing a blood clot in your legs.)

GETTING IN SHAPE

In the world of physical activity, if walking is the meat and potatoes, then exercise is the dessert. It completes the meal, so to speak.

The best way to exercise is by doing exactly what our guests at Pritikin do: combine aerobic, resistive, and stretching exercises *that you enjoy*. We cannot stress this enough. The more enjoyment you get from your activities, the more likely you are to stick with them. If you hate running, then definitely don't take up jogging! But if you love tennis and golf, as I do, find a way to maximize your time playing them. A gentle yoga class that nourishes you physically and spiritually is a far better option for you than a high-intensity hip-hop class that leaves you frustrated and limping. Another person may love that same hip-hop class and think your yoga session is a big snooze, but remember, you have to find what works best for *you*.

Just like Will Rogers, who never met a man he didn't like, the Pritikin Program likes all forms of physical activity. It is just that some activities are better than others. There is good reason to try to incorporate at least one type of each form of exercise into your routine. Keep reading.

Aerobic Exercise

Aerobic exercises, such as jogging, biking, stair climbing, hiking, swimming, tennis, and dancing, increase your heart rate and blood circulation and burn calories. Because it is the most strenuous form of physical activity, aerobic exercise is the best way to lower your blood pressure, cholesterol, weight, and risk of heart disease and stroke. This does not mean that walking isn't good for you; it just means that jogging prevents heart disease better.

I know what you're thinking: you can't jog or run very far. That's okay; I'm not asking you to. I want you to try this instead: Warm up, then stretch a little, and then jog or run at a good clip for one to two minutes. Then walk or jog slowly for a few minutes until you catch your breath. Again, jog or run quickly for another one to two minutes, then walk again for a few minutes. Keep alternating for 30 minutes, then cool off and stretch. You have just completed your first interval exercise. These peaks of high heart rate and blood circulation are of maximum benefit to your heart.

Unfortunately, most Americans who jog just do it slowly, for hours. Or worse, they buy expensive, computer-controlled treadmills and set them at a constant slow speed while they watch television or read. The treadmills actually have computerized brains in them that allow you to mimic walking or jogging up and down hills; use your own brain and program the computer for interval exercise.

Don't overdo the peak exercise portions when you first start doing interval exercise. Build up slowly, using your heart rate as your guide (see the text box on the next page for how to calculate your heart rate). If after the first peak, your heart rate is more than 90 percent of your maximum, you overshot your goal. If your heart rate is below 75 percent of your maximum, try jogging or running faster on the next peak portion. You will find that you will gradually become more comfortable at faster peak rates; this is a sign that you are increasing your fitness.

Calculating Your Heart Rate

Your heart rate is a reasonable estimate of how much aerobic exercise you are doing. Your resting heart rate should be between 60 and 80 beats per minute. Your *maximum heart rate* is about 220 minus your age (though there is some variation from person to person). Good aerobic exercise gets your heart rate up to at least 75 percent of your maximum, but no more than 90 percent. For example, if you are 60 years old, your maximum heart rate is 160 beats per minute (220 minus 60). Ideally, you want your heart rate somewhere between 120 and 144 beats per minute (75%–90% of 160).

To count your beats per minute, check your pulse for about 15 seconds and multiply by four. If counting your pulse manually is difficult, buy a wrist, chest, or finger gauge that does it automatically.

Exercise Frequency: How often should you exercise? Countless studies have shown that more frequent exercise is better for us. It keeps us physically fit (two weeks without exercise almost eliminates your physical conditioning) and allows us to burn more calories even after we have stopped exercising (metabolism increases 8 to 28 percent after strenuous exercise for up to eight hours). Exercising strenuously only occasionally increases your risk of physical injury, not to mention heart attacks. A consistent routine of strenuous exercise two to three times per week at minimum keeps your triglycerides lowered, as the effect lasts about two days. I'd like to see everyone reading this book commit to at least 200 minutes of exercise per week, ideally divided into seven 30-minute episodes.

Exercise Duration: I don't think you were surprised when I recommended more frequent and more strenuous exercise. But the next statement might surprise you. Per episode of exercise, *you do not need to exercise* *for any more than 30 minutes.* You don't help your heart any more by running for an hour than you do for 30 minutes. Although you may burn more calories by exercising longer, you will probably exercise more strenuously by doing it for a shorter time, especially if you employ interval exercise. To put it another way, I'd rather see you work out harder than longer.

If you're currently exercising once or twice a week for an hour or more, I want you to change your pattern to five to seven times a week for 30 minutes. Even 20 minutes will do if you get your heart really pumping.

Resistive Exercise

Resistive exercise, such as weight lifting, builds lean muscle mass, which in turn decreases blood sugar and strengthens bones. Increasing your lean muscle mass increases your metabolic rate slightly—you can eat 100 more calories per day without gaining weight. It is also one of the best ways to prevent diabetes. Besides, the toning of your arms, legs, backside, and torso creates great visual results!

Resistive exercise can be done at home against gravity, such as push-ups, sit-ups, leg raises, and pull-ups, or with free weights or machines at home or the gym. See the Appendix A for the 10 simple resistive exercises we teach at the Pritikin Longevity Center.

Stretching

Flexibility exercises like stretching prevent muscle injury and strengthen your joints. Since both aerobic and resistive exercises shorten and tighten your muscles, adding stretching to your routine after you exercise is a good idea.

You don't want to stretch vigorously before you warm up. Jump in place or jog for a few minutes before you stretch seriously so that blood can begin flowing to your muscles. See Appendix B for the full-body stretching routine we use at Pritikin.

KEY POINTS TO REMEMBER

- Walking is a key component of a healthy lifestyle.
- A complete exercise program includes walking, aerobic exercise, resistive training, and stretching.
- Adequate aerobic exercise should increase your heart rate to at least 75 percent of your maximum heart rate (maximum heart rate = 220 minus your age).
- More frequent exercise is better.
- Strenuous exercise in shorter durations is better than lighter exercise for longer durations.
- Resistive exercise is beneficial because it increases lean muscle mass, decreases diabetes, and strengthens bones.
- Stretching is beneficial for protecting muscles and joints.

11

Pritikin Essential Ingredient 7: Go Lean on Meat, but Catch a Fish

CLASSICALLY, THERE HAVE been two good diets on earth to prevent heart disease, and unfortunately, the American diet isn't one of them. The two lucky regions were the southern Mediterranean and the Pacific Rim, epitomized by Greece, southern France, Italy, and Japan. Food in these fortunate cultures was generally delicious, healthful, and plentiful. Heart disease in these regions occurred much less frequently than in America, even at the same cholesterol levels. The "French Paradox" refers to this surprisingly low rate of heart disease despite high consumption of saturated fat. Unfortunately, the previously healthy diets in these cultures are catching up with ours, and so is their heart disease. And the French may not have had low rates of heart disease after all. Statisticians have found that the French are far more likely than other countries to classify sudden deaths not as heart disease, but from "sudden unknown causes."

What were the Greeks, Italians, French, and Japanese doing right 50 years ago, and what are we here in America doing wrong? Well, they had several dietary practices that were right in line with some of the Pritikin essentials you've already learned: they ate more fruits, vegetables, and whole grains, and less refined calorie-dense foods. They also did one other thing, which is the basis of Pritikin essential 7: they ate far less bad fats, such as those found in corn-raised red meat, and more good fats, such as those found in fish.

Several studies have compared heart disease rates in different cultures. One consensus observation is that the different rates of heart disease can be best explained by two factors: the types of fats and the amount of fruits and vegetables they consume. We have already covered the wonderful benefits of fruits and vegetables. Now let's tackle the complex world of fats. One of the best surveys is Ancel Key's Seven Countries Study, which compared fat intake, cholesterol, and heart disease in selected countries around the world after World War II. Here is what they found:

- During that era, Finland had the highest rate of heart disease, though the United States was not all that far behind. The saturated fats in red meats and whole milk products were the major culprits.
- The Finns, who ate an average of 20 percent of their calories as saturated fat, had 10 times the rate of heart disease as the Japanese, who ate only 5 percent of their calories as saturated fat (as well as higher quantities of fruits and vegetables). The Finns also had an average cholesterol level of nearly twice that of the Japanese.
- At the same time that the Finns were eating meat and cheese, the Greenland Eskimos were eating a daily average of one pound of fish. Unlike meat, fish is low in saturated fat and high in omega-3 fat (we'll get to what all these different types of fats mean in a moment). The Greenland Eskimos' lifetime risk for heart disease was only 3 percent—even lower than that of the heart-healthy Japanese. The Finnish high saturated fat diet caused 20 times more heart disease than the Eskimo high omega-3 fat diet. Genes did

not account for the difference; Eskimos living in Finland ate less fish and had a similar heart disease rate to the Finns.

So what does all this tell us? In a nutshell, that the type fat you eat matters.

THE DIFFERENT TYPES OF FATS

When it comes to acquiring or preventing heart disease, dietary fat is a key ingredient. Which fats you choose, and how often, will absolutely play a role. And, as with any lifestyle change, it's best to start with a clear understanding of the facts.

There are five major classes of fats:

- *Trans fats*, made from the partial hydrogenation of vegetable oils, found in margarines, pastries, fried foods, and many packaged foods.
- *Saturated fats*, found in meat, cheese, whole milk, and tropical oils.
- *Monounsaturated fats*, found in olives, avocados, and many nuts.
- *Omega-6 polyunsaturated fats*, found in many vegetable oils and some nuts.
- *Omega-3 polyunsaturated fats*, found in large amounts in fish and flaxseeds and in moderate amounts in rapeseeds, walnuts, soybeans, and pumpkin seeds.

What makes one fat different from another? It comes down to chemistry. All fats—really called "fatty acids"—are made up of a long chain of carbons. Visualize them as pearls on a string. What differentiates one fat from another is the length of the chain and the number of double bonds between the carbons; in other words, how many pearls on the strand are connected by a double string. Saturated fats have no double bonds, monounsaturated fats have one, and polyunsaturated fats have two or more. Omega-3 polyunsaturated fats have the most, with between three and six double bonds.

Something worth noting here is that vegetable origin does not necessarily signify good fat. The tropical oils, such as palm, palm kernel, and coconut oil, contain considerable saturated fat and very little omega-3s and are as bad for your arteries as butter and lard. Polynesians who eat considerable quantities of coconut oil have very high cholesterol levels. Fats from most domesticated animals are generally high in saturated fat and low in omega-3s. Fish fats, in contrast, are generally high in omega-3s and low in saturated fat.

Eating Less Saturated and Trans Fats

Saturated fat is the gold standard for heart-unhealthy food. It increases LDL (bad) cholesterol, inflammation, and clotting and decreases nitric oxide production—all major contributors to heart disease. Foods that are typically high in saturated fat include meat, cheese, whole-milk products, and tropical oils. Dietary saturated fat, not cholesterol, is the major cause of high blood cholesterol and especially high LDL (bad) cholesterol in most people. Low-cholesterol foods are not necessarily low in saturated fat. Coconuts have no cholesterol but are higher in saturated fat than cream cheese. A few foods, including shrimp and squid (calamari), have plenty of cholesterol but not much saturated fat. Some foods used to be labeled "low cholesterol" to masquerade their high saturated fat content, but the FDA no longer allows that.

Although there is no need to eat saturated fats, they are virtually impossible to totally exclude in a nutritionally adequate diet. Ideally, you want to eat no more than 5 to 10 grams of saturated fat per day. Our guests at the Pritikin Longevity Center average less than 10 grams per day. The saturated fat content of packaged foods is listed in the nutrition box; remember that the listing is per serving, not per container. Here are some suggestions and substitutions to reduce dietary saturated fats:

- Eat less red meat and dark-meat poultry.
- Change from fatty red meats to much leaner meats like skinless white-meat poultry and, especially, fish.
- Change from 1%, 2%, and whole-milk products (milk, cheese,

and ice cream) to fat-free milk products (skim milk, fat-free yogurt and frozen yogurt, and nonfat ricotta cheese).

- Avoid palm, palm kernel, and coconut oils in packaged foods.

Attention, Dieters!

Even on a low-carbohydrate diet, saturated fat is harmful. Bacon is still bacon.

If saturated fat is the gold standard for heart-unhealthy food, trans fat is the platinum standard. Trans fats found in pastries, some margarines, fried foods, and many snack and convenience foods are even worse than saturated fats ounce for ounce because they both raise LDL (bad) cholesterol and reduce HDL (good) cholesterol. Fortunately, we have in recent years begun eating less trans fat, but really, we should eat *no* trans fat. Starting in 2006, trans fat content is listed in the nutrition box on packaged foods, which has thankfully inspired many food companies to stop using trans fats (though knowing the altruism of the American food industry, we are probably going to see a resurgence in the use of almost-as-deadly tropical "vegetable" oils loaded with saturated fat). New York and other cities have recently banned trans fat in restaurants. The following foods are high in trans fats and should be avoided:

- commercial baked goods
- fried foods
- most crackers
- fast-food French fries and chicken
- biscuit mixes
- many types of candy
- microwave popcorn
- most doughnuts and other fried pastries
- most chips, corn puffs, and other snack junk foods

If reading the above list has left you wondering what's left to snack on, go back and reread Chapter 8, "Snack Smarter." There you'll find plenty of terrific options without deadly trans fats weighing them—and you—down.

Monounsaturated: The "Neutral" Fat

Smack in the middle of the spectrum are monounsaturated fats, which we consider "neutral" on cholesterol, but like all oils are packed with calories. They aren't the worst fats you can eat—clearly, saturated and trans fats take the prize for that—but they aren't the good "essential fats," either. Examples of foods containing monounsaturated fats are olives, avocados, and many nuts. Perhaps the monounsaturated fat that gets the star treatment of late is olive oil, but we have a few things we want you to know and understand about that before you buy into the marketing hype.

Olive oil has come into favor over the past few decades as the oil of choice, mostly because of its marketed associations with heart-healthy cultures like Italy. However, when it comes to choosing the best fats, scientific trials support the fact that olive oil in fact isn't at the top of the list—canola oil and similar omega-3–rich oils are.

All naturally occurring oils are mixtures of different types of fats. For example, olive oil is 78 percent monounsaturated fat, but also contains about 14 percent unhealthy saturated fat, 7 percent polyunsaturated fat, and less than 1 percent very healthy omega-3 fat. By contrast, canola oil contains slightly less monounsaturated fat (62 percent), but less than one-half as much saturated fat (6 percent) and 10 times as much omega-3 fat as olive oil. You would need to consume 10 times as much olive as canola oil to get the same amount of omega-3 fat. Unfortunately, that amount of olive oil would contain *30 times as much saturated fat—and 10 times more calories!*

Our laboratory at the University of Maryland has shown that typical olive oil reduces the protective nitric oxide, but typical canola oil does not. Certain olive oils, characterized by high antioxidant content, do not reduce nitric oxide, but these cannot be identified by their labels. "Extra-virgin" may sound very healthy, but it has nothing to do with antioxidant content. "Cold-pressed" is a healthier factor, since it is generally less oxidized, but even that label is not a guarantee that the oil is rich in antioxidants.

Admittedly, olive oil tastes good, especially on a salad. But a salad drenched in olive oil is neither slimming nor healthful. To me, a dash of canola or walnut oil mixed with several times as much balsamic vinegar tastes as good or better.

Cooking with canola oil is also preferable because canola oil oxidizes less than olive oil at high temperatures, but please avoid frying as much as possible. Even healthy foods fried in good oil should be avoided. High-temperature cooking and frying creates oxidized fats and end products that promote cardiovascular disease and diabetes. Reusing cooking oil is especially bad. Foods fried in used oil reduce nitric oxide even more than those fried in fresh oil. Limit the amount of fried foods you eat, but if you must fry, use fresh "high-temperature" canola oil.

Omega-3 Fats

Omega-3 fats, with the most double bonds (three to six), are the healthiest because they reduce inflammation, decrease heart rhythm disturbances, and reduce blood clotting (much like aspirin). Also, they do not reduce nitric oxide, as do most other fats. Omega-3 and omega-6 fats are dietary essentials, since we cannot synthesize them ourselves. Mostly, however, we believe that they are healthy because several prospective randomized trials show that they reduce the risk of heart attack and the chance of dying of heart disease.

Although omega-3 fats are the healthiest, there is honest debate about which food is the best source of these fats. Is it canola oil? Flaxseed oil? Fish? This isn't a question with a simple answer. Certain logic dictates that flaxseed oil is best (based on its 40 to 50 percent content of omega-3 fats), but other logic favors canola oil (used in the study with the greatest decrease in mortality, the Lyon Diet Heart study). Fish oil has more double bonds (four or six) than plant omega-3s (three), but dining from the deep has downsides as well, such as cost, mercury, and other potential toxins. Neither life nor science is easy; the best you can do is make as informed choices as possible and enjoy good fats in moderation, especially if you are trying to lose weight.

Fish, nuts, and oils are not the only sources of omega-3 fats. Small amounts of these fats are also found in vegetables, especially the green leafy variety, and beans. Omega-3 fats can even be obtained from the eggs of hens fed flaxseed meal, but egg yolks are still high in cholesterol, so they're not a good choice if you're seeking to reduce heart disease. The egg whites, with no fat, are okay in moderation.

Based on several studies of omega-3 fats, we recommend that you consume at least one to two grams of omega-3 fat per day. Sources of one gram of omega-3 include:

- Two to three ounces of salmon (wild is better than farmed)
- Two teaspoons of canola oil
- One teaspoon of ground flaxseeds
- Two teaspoons of pumpkin seeds
- Three one-gram over-the-counter fish oil capsules containing 30 percent omega-3 (not cod liver oil)
- One single-gram prescription omega-3 capsule (available through your doctor)

For losing weight, choose the seafood over the very calorie-dense oils. Two little teaspoons of oil pack in 83 calories.

Fishing for the Right Seafood

At Pritikin, we have a saying, "Go lean on meat, but catch a fish." Because fish is such a primary source of omega-3s, it can be part of a healthy, low-fat meal. We encourage you to incorporate it into your diet, but in moderation when it comes to those large predatory fish such as tuna and swordfish that have higher mercury levels.

Below are the ratings for many selections of fish, which includes how much healthy omega-3 fats, unhealthy saturated fats, cholesterol, salt, and mercury each contains. The ratings are based on the latest information from the USDA Nutrient Database, U.S. Environmental Protection Agency, and U.S. Food and Drug Administration. All ratings, unless otherwise noted, arc based on cooked, 3½-ounce servings.

A Great Catch

The following selections are high in omega-3s and low in saturated fat, cholesterol, salt, and mercury. Enjoy these fish often, up to one serving daily.

	Omega-3s (grams)	Saturated Fat (grams)	Cholesterol (mg)	Mercury (parts per million)	Sodium (mg)
Horring	2.0	2.6	77	.04	114
Mackerel (canned, no salt)	2.5	2.7	65	0.3	50
Mussels	0.8	0.9	56	None detected	369
Oysters	0.6	0.6	49	None detected	243
Salmon (canned, no salt)	1.6	1.5	55	None detected	75
Salmon (fresh, farmed)	1.4	1.9	63	None detected	52
Salmon (fresh, wild)	1.8	1.3	71	.01	56
Sardines (water-dense, no salt)	1.0	1.5	81	.02	45
Trout (farmed)	1.1	2.1	68	.03	42
Whitefish	1.6	1.2	77	.07	65

A Good Catch

Not as high in omega-3s, but still fairly low in saturated fat, cholesterol, salt, and mercury. Enjoy these fish, but when you can, choose "A Great Catch" first.

	Omega-3s (grams)	Saturated Fat (grams)	Cholesterol (mg)	Mercury (parts per million)	Sodium (mg)
Calamari (Squid)*	0.5	0.4	231	.07	44
Catfish (farmed)	0.2	1.8	64	.07	80
Catfish (wild)	0.2	0.7	72	.05	50
Clams	0.3	0.2	67	None detected	111
Cod	0.2	0.2	55	.11	78
Crabs: Dungeness (fresh)	0.4	0.2	76	.18	378
Crabs: Stone (fresh)	0.4	0.2	75	.18	370
Haddock	0.2	0.2	74	.03	87
Lobster: Florida	0.5	0.3	90	.09	226
Mahi Mahi (Dolphin)	0.1	0.2	94	.19	113
Pollock	0.5	0.2	90	.06	109
Scallops (6 ounces, raw)	0.4	0.1	53	.05	265
Shrimp*	0.3	0.3	194	None detected	223
Snapper	0.3	0.4	47	.19	57
Sole/ Flounder	0.5	0.4	68	.04	105
Tilapia	0.1	0.5	55	.01	60
Tuna (canned, light, in water, without salt)	0.3	0.2	30	.12	50

* Individuals with higher cholesterol levels should limit calamari and shrimp to one to two servings monthly.

A So-So Catch

Moderately high in mercury, so limit to one to two servings per month.

	Omega-3s (grams)	Saturated Fat (grams)	Cholesterol (mg)	Mercury (parts per million)	Sodium (mg)
Bluefish	1.0	1.2	76	.31	77
Crab: Alaska king (fresh)*	0.4	0.1	53	.06	1066
Halibut	0.5	0.4	41	.26	69
Lobster, Maine	0.1	0.1	72	.31	378
Sea Bass	1.0	0.7	102	.27	88
Trout (wild)	1.2	1.6	69	.27	56
Tuna: Albacore (canned, "white," in water, without salt)	0.9	0.8	42	.35	50
Tuna: Albacore (fresh)	0.9	0.9	42	.38	47
Tuna: Bluefin	1.5	1.6	49	.32	50
Tuna: Yellowfin	0.3	0.3	58	.33	37

* Though low in mercury, Alaska king crab is very high in salt. That's why it is "a so-so catch."

Throw It Back

High in mercury. Avoid these fish as much as possible.

	Omega-3s (grams)	Saturated Fat (grams)	Cholesterol (mg)	Mercury (parts per million)	Sodium (mg)
Grouper	0.2	0.3	47	.55	53
King Mackerel	NA	0.4	68	.73	203
Marlin	NA	NA	NA	.49	NA
Orange Roughy	0.0	0.0	26	.54	81
Shark	NA	0.9	51	.99	79
Swordfish	NA	1.4	50	.97	115
Tilefish	NA	0.8	64	1.5	59

Cholesterol

When you hear the word *cholesterol*, it is referring to one of two sorts: *blood cholesterol*, which is made in your liver (and is the number you're likely looking to lower if you're reading this book), and *dietary cholesterol*. About 10 to 15 percent of blood cholesterol comes from the cholesterol in the food you eat. If we eat too much cholesterol, we can raise our blood cholesterol somewhat, but what really sends our blood cholesterol soaring is saturated fat.

Major sources of dietary cholesterol are egg yolks, meats (including poultry), and whole-milk products. Egg whites are rich in protein and contain no cholesterol; fruits, nuts, and vegetables do not contain cholesterol either. Nonfat dairy products such as skim milk contain much less cholesterol than whole milk and have almost no saturated fat, so they're okay in moderation. Nearly all animal foods contain cholesterol, including fish and shellfish, so enjoy those in moderation, as well. Limiting daily cholesterol intake to less than 200 milligrams is a starting recommendation. At the Pritikin Center, we recommend even less than that—ideally no more than 100 milligrams per day and even less for those trying to reverse heart disease.

Here are some basic guidelines for cholesterol levels in common foods:

1 jumbo egg (yolk)	270 mg	skim milk (8 oz)	4 mg
liver (4 oz)	450 mg	whole milk (8 oz)	30 mg
beef (4 oz)	100 mg	cheese (1 oz)	30 mg
chicken (4 oz)	100 mg	ice cream (4 oz)	50 mg
turkey (4 oz)	120 mg	butter (1 tbsp)	30 mg
salmon (4 oz)	70 mg	nonfat yogurt (8 oz)	4 mg
tuna (4 oz)	40 mg	fruits, nuts, vegetables	0 mg
shrimp or squid (4 oz)	200 mg	grains, beans	0 mg

Several foods, such as beans, soluble fiber-rich fruits, vegetables, oats, barley, and soy products actually lower blood cholesterol. They are important ingredients in a heart-healthy diet, although some, like soy products, are calorie-dense, so go easy on them if you're trying to lose weight. The fact that some fatty foods, such as certain margarines with plant sterols, can lower blood cholesterol may be surprising. But a recent study demonstrated that a diet containing the combination of nuts (1 ounce), soy protein (1.5 ounces), soluble fiber (20 grams), and margarine containing plant sterol (2 grams) reduced LDL (bad) cholesterol by 29 percent—just as much as a cholesterol-lowering medication. Sterols and stanols are plant-derived additives in several commercially available margarines, such as Benecol and Promise's Take Control, and one brand of orange juice (Minute Maid Heart Wise). Unfortunately, nuts, margarine, and soy products are calorie-dense. We at Pritikin recommend plant sterol supplements like Cholest-Off, which don't have the extra calories.

Do not sell short the beneficial effects of certain foods; healthy eating means adding good foods as much as avoiding bad foods. Here are five foods, all of which can lower your cholesterol by 5 to 10 percent if consumed daily for three to four weeks:

- 1 tablespoon stanol/sterol canola oil margarine
- 50 grams soy protein
- 10 grams soluble fiber
- 3 ounces walnuts
- Two 1-gram plant sterol supplements

Let's take a look at each of these foods to figure out which ones can lower your cholesterol *and* your weight.

- 1 tablespoon stanol/sterol canola oil margarine (100 calories)
- 50 grams soy protein (at least 500 calories from soy foods)
- 10 grams soluble fiber (only about 25 calories from sugar-free Metamucil)
- 3 ounces walnuts (550 calories)

- Plant sterol supplements (0 calories—this is one of the rare instances where supplements are better than food)

Margarines: Margarine is an excellent example of a food that can be very bad or somewhat good. Some trans fat rich margarines are every bit as bad for your heart as butter. Generally, the harder stick margarines that contain hydrogenated oils have the most trans fats, and should be avoided. Soft tub margarines made from safflower, sunflower, and corn oils contain reasonable amounts of polyunsaturated fats and less trans fats—these margarines are clearly better than butter. Softer tub margarines made from canola oil are even better, because they contain about 10 percent omega-3 fat and are low in saturated fat.

The best margarines, if you must use one, are made from canola oil and contain added plant stanols or sterols. Examples are Benecol and Take Control. These plant stanols and sterols are cholesterol-related molecules that can block the absorption of cholesterol in the intestines. Stanols and sterols are "natural" in that they are found in foods such as nuts, seeds, whole grains, beans, fruits, and vegetables. Two to three tablespoons of these plant sterol–enriched margarines lower LDL (bad) cholesterol 10 to 15 percent and supply three grams of omega-3 fat.

If you are a butter or margarine user, changing to these margarines is a no-brainer. If you are going to use some spread, it might as well be one with some health pluses. The plant sterol-enriched margarines can also be used in cooking. A baked sweet potato topped with a tablespoon of enriched margarine lowers your cholesterol as much as fast-food French fries raise it.

Remember, the calories of the best margarines do add up, and obesity itself raises your cholesterol. That can be a problem. Plant sterol margarines add almost as many calories to your diet as butter: each tablespoon contains 100 calories. We don't serve them at the Pritikin Longevity Center, since most people there are trying to lose weight. If you're trying to lose weight, keep your daily intake to one teaspoon or less of these heart-healthful but calorie-dense margarines.

Nuts: One of the most underrated high-fat foods is nuts. Many nuts contain natural cholesterol absorption-blocking sterols. The most heart-healthy nuts are walnuts and almonds, but most nuts are good sources of omega-3 and other polyunsaturated fats and fat-soluble vitamins. Peanuts, which are legumes rather than true nuts, may also have health benefits. Being unrefined and unprocessed, the unsalted varieties of nuts make excellent snacks, *but only in small portions*. Three ounces of walnuts per day reduce cholesterol about 10 percent, but contain about *500 calories*! Nuts are calorie-dense, so if your goal is weight loss, be careful. An ounce every day would add up to 17.5 extra pounds in one year.

The science is there to back up nuts' ability to reduce heart disease. People who ate nuts as part of a comprehensive diet plan in the Indo-Mediterranean Diet Study had 40 percent fewer heart attacks. One observational study showed that women who eat peanut butter have less diabetes than those who don't. Almond butter might be even better.

KEY POINTS TO REMEMBER

- Be sure to get enough healthy, essential fats like omega-3s.
- Lower your intake of saturated fats as much as possible.
- Do not eat foods containing trans fats.
- Enjoy even the healthier fats in moderation if you are trying to lose weight.
- Restrict your dietary cholesterol to less than 100 milligrams per day.

12

Pritikin Essential Ingredient 8: Shake Your Salt Habit

IN 2005, NUTRITION expert Dr. Stephen Havas at the University of Maryland School of Medicine said, "The number of deaths that occur because we eat too much salt is equivalent to a jumbo jet crashing every single day." Actually, we believe it's closer to two jumbo jets—that's how dangerous are the repercussions of eating too much salt.

What's so bad about salt, you might ask? Well, salt in our diets is a direct cause of high blood pressure (hypertension), which is the most common cardiovascular disease in the United States. Recent research has found that at least 90 percent of all citizens can expect to be diagnosed with hypertension during their lifetime. And the risks don't end there: the higher your blood pressure, the higher your risk of stroke, heart attack, congestive heart failure, kidney disease, and even dementia.

Hypertension results from increased resistance to blood flow and/or increased blood volume that forces the heart to work harder and at higher pressures than normal to push more blood through circulation. A high salt intake increases blood volume because it holds on to water in the body; the increased blood volume increases blood pressure, much like adding air to a tire. Excess salt also constricts your arteries, impeding blood flow. The most insidious fact of hypertension, often called "the silent killer," is that it usually shows no symptoms until very late in the disease process, so over time, damage to the circulatory system can occur before the condition is ever diagnosed. Your first symptom could be a stroke or heart attack. That's why it is so important to have your blood pressure checked regularly, and to reduce your salt intake now before it is too late.

Do I Have High Blood Pressure?

Blood pressure measurements, obtained using a blood pressure cuff, contain two numbers: the first number (the top one) is the *systolic* pressure, or the pressure in the arteries when the heart contracts. The second number (the bottom one) is the *diastolic* pressure, which refers to pressure in the arteries when the heart is relaxing and filling with blood.

So, what does *your* blood pressure measurement mean? Here are the ranges:

- Optimal blood pressure is no more than 110/70.
- Normal blood pressure is less than 120/80.
- Borderline hypertension, or pre-hypertension, is between 120/80 and 140/90.
- Hypertension is blood pressure 140/90 or higher.

The science on high salt intake leading to high blood pressure is now so solid that the Institutes of Medicine—independent scientists who advise the government—cut the recommended sodium intake a few years ago from 2,400 milligrams a day to 1,500 milligrams or less. The average American ingests a whopping 4,000 milligrams a day.

If you're still not convinced that you need to reduce your salt intake, consider the landmark research done by the National Institutes of Health known as the DASH studies. It compared diets with varying levels of sodium (3,300, 2,400, and 1,500 milligrams a day) on more than 400 people and found that the biggest reductions in blood pressure for everyone—people with hypertension as well as those with low blood pressure readings—occurred in those consuming only 1,500 milligrams of sodium per day.

Moreover, the follow-up portion of the Trials of Hypertension Prevention published in 2007 found that salt reduction lowered cardiovascular disease by 25 percent.

Lowering your blood pressure starts with losing weight if you are overweight. Losing even 10 to 20 pounds can reduce your blood pressure significantly. By now, you should be well versed in the Pritikin essentials that will enable you to lose weight. Now let's talk about how you're going to actually reduce the salt in your diet that causes the high blood pressure in the first place.

REDUCING YOUR SALT INTAKE

We have a lot of experience at Pritikin in helping people normalize their blood pressure. Results published as early as 1983 showed that after just one month of following the Pritikin Program, more than 80 percent of patients with hypertension were able to discontinue their medication—and maintain a blood pressure as low as or lower than when they arrived. Since then, several other studies have documented that most people who entered the Pritikin Longevity Center with high blood pressure ended their three-week stay with normal blood pressure; in one analysis of 1,117 people with hypertension, more than half no longer required any blood pressure medication within one month of starting the Pritikin Program. Most of the rest had some blood pressure drugs eliminated and/or the doses reduced.

The change begins in our daily lectures and classes, where guests learn about the effects of salt and how much they should be ingesting (as opposed to how much they actually are!), and continues in our beautiful, sun-filled dining room as they learn that they really don't have to give up flavor because they're cutting back on sodium. There's a universe of seasonings Pritikin's creative chefs use to add zest to food. For seafood, they might use fresh dill and fresh lemon; for baby red potatoes, fresh rosemary and sage; for roasted chicken breast, fresh cilantro, fresh onion, and salsa. For your own cooking and tasting enjoyment, refer to the recipes that are included in Part Three.

The Stats on Sodium and Salt

Table salt is the chemical sodium chloride, whether it is sea salt, rock salt, iodized salt, or any other variety. Regardless of what form you choose, it is very easy to eat a lot of sodium with just a few jiggles of the salt shaker:

- One teaspoon of table salt = 6 grams of salt, or about 2,300 mg sodium
- One teaspoon of sea salt = 5 grams of salt, or 2,000 mg sodium
- One tablespoon soy sauce = 2.5 grams of salt, or about 1,000 mg sodium

Most Americans now consume 3,500 to 5,000 milligrams of sodium per day. Considering that our national guideline is between 1,200 and 1,500 milligrams per day—a guideline with which the Pritikin Program fully agrees—we need to make some changes to what we're eating, and fast.

Daily Sodium Guidelines

The Institute of Medicine, comprised of the country's leading researchers in health and nutrition, issued the following guidelines for daily sodium consumption:

(continued)

- People ages 19 to 50 should consume 1,500 milligrams or less of sodium a day.
- People ages 51 to 69 should consume 1,300 milligrams or less.
- People over 70 should consume 1,200 milligrams or less.

Eating Well on a Low-Sodium Diet

We know what you're thinking: food without salt tastes terrible. But bear with us, please! We've helped millions of people worldwide kick their high-salt habit, and we can help you, too. Remember, our tastes buds can get used to anything in time; it's exactly the same when we switch from whole milk to skim, regular soda to diet, sugar to no-calorie sweetener.

At Pritikin, many of our guests experience for the first time the subtler, natural flavors of foods not saturated with salt. For some, it's not an easy lesson to learn, because excess salt dulls our taste buds. The first day or two, they're grumbling to our chefs: "Did you forget to put the seasonings in the Chinese Tomato Soup?" But then, just five to six days later, they're accusing the chefs of slipping salt into the soup because "it's just too flavorful." That's how quickly our taste for salt can change.

What's wonderful, too, is that once people's "bliss point" or "just right" amount of salt is lowered, they're turned off by salty foods. In fact, many, like longtime Pritikin alum Leonard Riggio, founder and chairman of Barnes & Noble, Inc., said, "I absolutely do not like the taste of salt anymore." What they do love are the many rich flavors of fresh herbs like basil and rosemary, and seasoning blends like herbes de Provence.

It's a whole new world once you're rid of the salt habit. Many Americans may think Doritos are the ultimate afternoon snack, but Leonard Riggio declares they don't even come close to a mango. "Just think about the taste. A mango *explodes* in your mouth," he enthuses. "Even better are 'm and m's,' and we're not talking candy. Mint and mango, that's *the* flavor combination." Leonard breaks the mint leaves, squeezes out the mint oil, and rubs it over the mango, surrounding the mango with the essence of mint.

This isn't self-sacrifice. It's self-indulgence! Your taste buds have come alive again.

So how can you reduce the amount of salt in your diet and experience a whole new range of taste sensations? Here are some tips:

- Pick packaged foods with fewer milligrams of sodium than calories. Avoid high-salt canned soups, most packaged breads, processed meats, chips, sauces, et cetera. Seek out lower-sodium alternatives, or, in the case of soups, make your own (see the recipes in Part Three).
- Insist on no added salt at restaurants, and limit or avoid most soups and sauces.
- Do not put salt or salty condiments, like soy sauce, on the table. If they aren't there, you will be less tempted to use them. If you like the taste of soy sauce, try less-sodium varieties, but don't go overboard. One tablespoon of less-sodium soy sauce still has 575 mg of sodium.
- Avoid salt-rich seasonings, such as garlic salt and onion salt, in cooking
- Avoid fast food; it is extremely high in salt.
- Stick to natural, whole foods; they contain little salt.
- Learn to spice up food without salt or with just a little. Experiment with other seasonings, lemon juice, fresh herbs, and balsamic vinegar. There are many wonderful recipes in Part Three that will teach you how to season without salt so your food tastes delicious.

KEY POINTS TO REMEMBER

- High blood pressure can result in stroke, heart disease, and kidney failure.
- Reducing your salt intake directly lowers your blood pressure.
- The ideal daily range of sodium intake is no more than 1,200 to 1,500 milligrams, depending on age.
- Our taste buds can, and will, quickly adjust to a lower-sodium diet—and once they do, you'll taste food in a whole new way.

13

Pritikin Essential Ingredient 9: Don't Smoke Your Life Away

THIS CHAPTER IS as important as it is short. Cigarette smoking kills 435,000 Americans prematurely every year. That toll is more than the number of American soldiers killed during the four years of World War II. Even after years of high-profile public health campaigns, smoking remains the leading cause of preventable premature death in the United States. About 24 percent of adult Americans still smoke; that number has held relatively steady for the past decade. Sadly, though, the teenage smoking rate has increased from 29 percent to 35 percent.

Cigarette smoking causes heart attacks, strokes, cancer, emphysema, amputations, and sudden death. Smoking causes cardiovascular disease, because it injures your endothelium and decreases HDL (good) cholesterol and nitric oxide (pipes and cigars are almost as deadly for your heart as cigarettes, and their consequence—head and neck cancer— is an awful disease). Smoking injures the people around you through passive smoke inhalation, which is almost as deadly as smoking itself.

Remember how heart disease is a community concern? Well, so is smoking. It depletes our health-care resources, and those who smoke are making it far more likely that their children will smoke, perpetuating the problem.

Facts About Smoking

- You lose one minute of life for every minute you spend smoking.
- You lose two and a half hours of life per pack of cigarettes, and seven or eight years if you continue to smoke, or 10 percent of your life.
- If you stop smoking at age 30, you will restore four to five years of life.
- If you stop smoking at age 60, you will restore one to two years of life.

After I have told my patients everything above, I tell my male patients that smoking can make them impotent, which is true, and I tell my female patients that smoking will give them wrinkles, which is also true. Many seem to care more about those issues than they do about death, heart disease, stroke, cancer, and being tethered to an oxygen tank. But if sex and/or vanity will make them stop smoking, I'm all for it.

Knowing everything that we do about smoking, why do people still smoke? Kids start smoking to look mature, as a result of peer pressure, to rebel, or just to experiment. Many kids try smoking because they like dangerous and antisocial behavior; then they get hooked, sometimes after just one pack of cigarettes. Habits are hard to break, but addictions are even harder. Adults smoke for all kinds of bad reasons: to deal with stress, to control weight, to accompany drinking or eating, or just to feel good. The biological reasons are habituation and nicotine addiction.

If you smoke, please read the consequences I outlined here over and over, keeping your family and friends in mind. Then talk to your doctor about the antidepressant bupropion, nicotine patches and gum, and a new drug, varenicline, that can help you stop smoking. After doing all that, register for a smoking cessation program. We have a wonderful and effective program at the Pritikin Longevity Center & Spa. Programmatic support combined with medication is the most effective way to stop smoking.

If you decide not to quit smoking, good luck explaining to yourself and those who love you why you are choosing to shorten your life.

KEY POINTS TO REMEMBER

- Every minute spent smoking shortens your life by a minute.
- Smoking causes heart disease, strokes, cancer, and emphysema—not to mention impotence and wrinkles.
- Quitting smoking now can add years back to your life.
- Consult your doctor and/or a program that offers support for assistance with quitting.

14

Pritikin Essential Ingredient 10: Step Around Stress

STRESS IS WIDELY misunderstood in our culture. Stress is not simply unpleasant experiences or potentially harmful experiences or circumstances. A hectic life doesn't necessarily translate to a stressful one; unemployed people may be more stressed than busy CEOs. Stress is created by *how we react to these difficult circumstances*.

Take, for example, Dr. Dean Ornish's story of 11-year-old Tim and his father. One day last year Tim's father was driving him to a soccer meet, for which they were very late. As they pulled up to an intersection, the train lights started flashing and the gate came down, signaling the cars to stop to allow a slow freight train to pass through. Tim's father responded in frustration, "Damn, now we are going to be even later."

Innately, Tim responded, "Yeah, but now we get to see a great big freight train go by." His perception changed the whole event.

When we respond in a stressed fashion to unpleasant circumstances, we initiate the basic fight-or-flight physiology with which we are genetically encoded. Adrenaline and related hormones are quickly released; heart rate, blood pressure, blood sugar, inflammation, and blood clotting increase as a result. Why? Because our bodies were designed to become stronger, bleed less, and repair damage more quickly during and after fights with wild animals. Fortunately, such stressful circumstances rarely occur today. Unfortunately, though, "fights" with fellow drivers, bosses, spouses, and kids occur all the time. Our bodies still respond the same way to these new hostilities.

If stress continues, the slower-acting hormone cortisol is released. Like adrenaline, cortisol increases blood pressure and sugar. Fat deposits within the abdomen increase, leading to metabolic syndrome and diabetes. By increasing blood pressure, inflammation, and clotting, stress also accelerates atherosclerosis.

Does Stress Really Cause Heart Attacks?

The short answer is yes, both directly through an increase in the factors that promote atherosclerosis and indirectly through its emotional effects. Studies have shown that earthquakes and Mondays double the incidence of heart attacks, and that heart disease kills men three times as frequently in the year following a wife's death.

THE SOURCES OF STRESS

Potentially stressful circumstances are all around us. Fear of harm is one of the most stressful circumstances. Besides the newly acquired threat of terrorism that we live with now, over the past 40 years we've seen violent crime rates quadruple, the prison population increase fivefold, and substance abuse increase eightfold. Even reading this paragraph causes stress! The Index of National Civilian Health, which measures personal and social well-being, has decreased 32 percent while our financial income has doubled. That's simply not a good trade-off, if you ask us.

Time Constraints

Time is often judged to be the most precious commodity in life. Yet none of us, it seems, has enough discretionary time; it's a major characteristic of the American lifestyle. If you ask 100 people how they are doing on any given day, we'd bet no fewer than 75 of them would respond, "Busy . . . so busy!" We're all rushing to and fro, constantly feeling pressured to get where we need to be. And even if we get there on time, there are still more things to do in a day, a month, a year than we could possibly have time for. Most people, like Tim's father in the story about the freight train, react to all these demands on their time in a stressful fashion.

Job Stress

Workplace stress is pervasive. As a nation, we rank third in productivity per hour, but we are the most productive people on Earth because we work the most hours. We have cannibalized time spent with our families and friends to make more work time. The signs that our increasing stress is taking a toll are all around us: divorce has doubled in the past 50 years, and the diagnosis of depression—a major sign of stress—has increased tenfold.

Volunteers in one study urged to perform arithmetic rapidly experienced an increase in blood pressure and a decrease in nitric oxide—two primary promoters of atherosclerosis. Volunteers asked to defend themselves from a false accusation of shoplifting had a measurable decrease in nitric oxide for as long as four hours after the event.

Like stress in general, job stress is often misunderstood. Stressed and busy occupations are not the same. Stressed occupations combine heavy psychological demands with a lack of options. On average, assembly-line workers are highly stressed; CEOs are moderately stressed, whereas foresters are only lightly stressed (though that might change during fire season).

Anger and Loneliness

Stress isn't the only heart-stopping emotion. Anger, frustration, tension, loneliness, and depression can also cause heart disease.

Physiologically, anger is very similar to stress. Heart disease patients are almost as likely to get chest pain when angry as when exercising. In a community study involving 130,000 subjects, anger-prone individuals developed heart disease twice as frequently as others over a five-year period. Coronary disease also progresses more rapidly in anger-prone people; those with low social support have three times faster progression of their artery narrowing compared with less angry individuals with good support around them.

Loneliness can take a toll on us emotionally and physically. Socially isolated people have a higher risk of heart disease. The death of a spouse and divorce are the two most stressful life events, and are followed by a period during which heart attacks and strokes occur three times as often. A recent 12-year, 9,000-subject British study found that government workers with poor close relationships had 34 percent more heart attacks. Socially isolated people also do not survive as well as others after heart attacks.

People differ in how much they need close relationships, but social isolation is nearly always a health hazard.

Images in the Media

Your head is connected to your heart when it comes to heart disease. Does entertainment have the same good and bad effects on heart disease as real life? Since entertainment is such a big part of the American lifestyle, a colleague of mine, Dr. Michael Miller, and I investigated the effect of watching violent and humorous videos on the nitric oxide levels of cardiology fellows in our hospital. Not surprisingly, those who watched the humorous videos produced more nitric oxide; those who watched violent war movies produced less. When it comes to emotional responses, your vascular system doesn't know the difference between violence and humor in real life and that which is in movies; your heart has the same emotional response whether you're watching it or actually living it.

STEPPING AROUND STRESS

Stressful circumstances cannot be totally eliminated. It isn't even necessary that we try to remove every source of stress in our lives; not all stresses are bad. For instance, any athlete knows that being "up" for competition improves performance. We are a socially and economically competitive society, so we sometimes need to be "up" in our daily lives. The problem is that *chronic and repetitive stress* cause heart disease.

Whenever possible, step around unnecessary stressful circumstances. If tardiness stresses you, leave plenty of time to get where you are going. If you are habitually out of time, don't put so much on your plate. If you know spending time with a certain person causes you stress or anxiety, try cutting back on the amount of time you spend with him or her. Limiting the number of stressful circumstances in your life is a small start.

And, when you cannot avoid stressful circumstances, the best way to step around stress is to learn how to respond better. A key component of stress reduction is adopting better perceptions (changing your outlook or the way you view a certain circumstance) and better ways of interacting with those who cause us stress. We call this taking an "emotionally nourishing" approach. When we get control of our lives in this way, we naturally feel less stressed.

STRESS REDUCTION TOOLS

To reduce the amount of stress in your life, adopt as many of the 10 activities listed below as possible; more enjoyment of life will be a welcome bonus.

- Become emotionally nourishing.
- Exercise regularly.
- Get sufficient sleep.
- Develop close relationships.
- Laugh.
- Touch others and enjoy a regular sexual relationship.
- Get a pet, especially a dog.
- Reserve time for enjoyable activities.
- Develop spiritually.
- Consider meditation, tai chi, and/or yoga.

Become Emotionally Nourishing

Your outlook is closely tied to your physical health. Emotionally nourishing people inspire a feast of joy in everyone around them. Sourpusses dine on meager emotional scraps. Emotionally nourishing people are those you would love to marry, have for a friend, or meet at a party. They make you smile inside and out.

The three essential ingredients of emotional nourishment are unconditional friendship and love, humor, and optimism. I would have used an existing word or phrase for this combination of healthy emotional qualities if one existed. In psychobabble, this kind of friendly, upbeat thinking is called positive cognitive restructuring. Pretty catchy, isn't it? Right. Joie de vivre comes close, but it is not exactly the same. Emotionally nourishing people initiate and amplify joy. During interactions, they respond in supportive, affirmative ways. They make others feel good just by being around them.

We all know emotionally nourishing people; we just may never have focused on how emotional nourishment makes our lives healthy as well as happy. Just as stress, anger, and social isolation accelerate heart disease, affection, optimism, and enjoyment of life retard it. We can help avoid heart disease by surrounding ourselves with humorous, friendly, loving people, and by coloring our own emotions in the same way.

CASE STUDY: THE POLISH POKER PLAYERS

My closest friends are a geographically dispersed collection of reprobate, curmudgeonly academic cardiologists and spouses who travel and teach cardiology in some of the nicest venues on Earth. My friend Jack assembled the group at his Snowmass meeting more than 30 years ago. Our favorite pastime is Polish poker. You need two hours or more, a lot of wine, and at least 10 friends to play. Twenty is even better. Everyone starts with three one-dollar bills. You get one card with each deal. Going around the table in turn, if you don't want your one card, you can exchange it with the person on your left, unless that person has a king. High card, starting with the queen, loses. Lose the hand and you forfeit one dollar to the pot. It's not intended to be a very cerebral game.

Cathy is the queen of the Polish poker players. A tall, emotionally nourishing Minnesotan, she is rarely without a smile on her face and open arms for a hug. Cathy recites the moronically simple rules each and every time we play. Everyone pretends to not understand. It is a ritual. We count on someone to have an extra dollar in his pot. We sing loudly whenever someone is busted after losing his or her last dollar. We get complaints from the neighbors. We love each other.

A few years ago, two of us convinced the Aspen Ski Corporation to name a run at Snowmass after Jack. His run, "Jack of Hearts," is a friendly, open slope, always well groomed, with nice bumps in all the right places. Ski it when you're there.

My wife, Sharyn, is the Polish poker players' photographer. Sharyn is an emotionally nourishing "domestic goddess." Her business card says so. I eat well, very well—by candlelight, enjoying fresh food cooked from scratch—every day. Can you eat very well every day in America and stay thin? You bet! My wife and I weigh 270 pounds . . . when we step on a scale at the same time. That's what this book is about.

Sharyn collects people like others collect knickknacks. Sharyn's second-favorite holiday is April Fool's Day. I have been tricked and made to look ridiculous in every way imaginable. My favorite episode occurred about 10 years ago on April Fool's eve. Sharyn and Sallie (the lovely gardener from

Chapter 4) traded places in the middle of the night without waking up either her husband or me. That morning, I didn't even have to get out of bed to get fooled. Clearly, such foolery is not for amateurs. Moreover, I do not recommend that you try such a stunt at home unless both husbands have had recent, completely normal stress tests.

A sequel to that episode proved to me that there is justice in this world. A year later, Sharyn was scheduled to pick up Sallie's daughter, Rachel, from school, but Sallie had forgotten to put her on the pickup list. The teacher would not let Rachel leave with my wife until the six-year-old suddenly and loudly announced to the class that it was okay because "Sharyn sleeps with my daddy." Problem solved. I could not make up that story.

We all have emotionally nourishing friends like those in my Polish poker–playing circle. They are the optimistic, social, and unconditionally affectionate people in our lives that make us happy just by being in their presence.

Make time for these people; your heart depends on it in more ways than one.

Change Your Inner Dialogue: If you are looking for a good source of optimism and affection, start with yourself. You probably spend more time talking with yourself than any other person. You wouldn't purposely seek out someone who was always putting you down, yet many people have a lifelong self-critical, pessimistic dialogue with themselves.

You must learn to become your own best friend. Let's start with a potentially stressful circumstance, such as losing a sales account. Here are typical examples of unproductive, self-critical inner dialogues that you'll want to recognize and reverse:

- "I'm going to get fired."
- "Bad things are always happening to me."
- "I can't do anything right."
- "I am a lousy salesman."

Add that subjective insult to the actual injury (if indeed there even was one) that spawned the negative chatter, and you have even more stress. Now, let's try a different approach:

- Start by giving some objective thought to *why* you lost the account. If you didn't do your homework, that's a lesson to prepare better the next time so you can be more successful. Analysis of the circumstance is productive; self-criticism is destructive.
- Instead of letting the loss of the sale get you down and projecting an "I can't do anything right" vibe to your boss (which he or she definitely won't appreciate and will likely lead to worse problems), give your boss an honest appraisal of what improvements you think need to be made in the sales process or product. Your boss will be impressed by your proactive response, and you'll feel good about yourself for turning it around.
- Keep things in proper perspective. You may have lost the sale, but your life is fundamentally good. You are healthy, you have a wonderful family, you have made a lot of big sales before—and you'll make others in the future.

Can you actually change your ongoing inner dialogue? Yes. Just as a negative inner dialogue leads to other self-criticism, a positive perspective on life propagates other upbeat thinking. We all know that we have good and bad emotional days. Stay with the positive thoughts, though, and other upbeat emotions will generally follow. It's all right to be self-critical at times, as long as you learn to balance your inner dialogue with positive thinking. Periodically, try making a list of all the good things going on in your life. Soon you will realize, just like 11-year-old Tim did earlier in this chapter, that you may be late, but you get to watch a really neat train go by.

Improve Your Interactions with Others: Would you rather interact with a warm, optimistic, nonjudgmental, polite, outgoing person or an unfriendly, critical, rude, terse one? No contest. Knowing that you'd rather have the former as a friend, colleague, spouse, or family member—and that all interactions between two people involve the energy of both parties—wouldn't it make sense to strive to become more emotionally nourishing to the people around you?

Just as with changing your inner dialogue, becoming more emotionally nourishing starts with positive perception and interaction. (All you happily married people out there probably know what I mean when I talk about "selectively positive interaction".) Here are a few tips to get you started improving your interactions with others to create harmony and emotional nourishment all the way around:

- Compliment whenever possible. Most of us respond better to praise than to criticism. If the meat loaf was great but the pie soggy, praise the meat loaf. Dwell on the pie at your own risk of paying for more take-out and restaurant meals. The cook already knows that the pie was soggy.

- Comment on actions, not personal qualities. If your child forgets to do his or her homework, do not blame it on stupidity. Your child will begin to believe the label and act accordingly, and will also label others as stupid whenever they fail.

- Give people the interaction for which they are asking. Be quiet and listen to a talkative or troubled friend. Laugh with a comic.

- Humor is therapeutic; use it to diffuse tense interactions.

- Fight fairly. It's easy to laugh with someone when times are good, but how we deal with conflict will determine long-term relations. Criticize the conduct, not the individual. Learn to accept and not continually criticize the faults of others that cannot or will not be changed.

- Do not threaten abandonment. Starting a marital argument with a threat of divorce is like going into a salary negotiation with a threat of quitting. You may win a raise or an argument, but your boss or spouse now knows that you want to leave.

- Provide others with what they really need. It is your responsibility to provide the material and nurturing needs of a home, school, or workplace. Emotionally nourishing people know the importance of being good providers, spouses, parents, and teachers.

Take Care of Yourself: A final word about becoming emotionally nourishing: lead a healthy lifestyle and take care of your appearance. All emotionally nourishing people are not necessarily physically beautiful, but they understand that their appearance and clothes project what they think of themselves.

Exercise Regularly

You already learned about the myriad of benefits exercise has on your physical health, but what about your overall well-being?

Most of my favorite ways to reduce stress involve exercise, with walking topping the list. Any day without exercise leaves me feeling wired. Most people, like me, are able to feel their stress levels fall with exercise. Even 30 minutes of walking dramatically reduces anxiety levels. Exactly how does physical activity reduce stress? Stress increases adrenaline, making the body ready for peak action. Exercise quenches that readiness for action. It literally takes the edge off.

Physical activity is generally as effective as any antidepressant drug. During exercise, your mind loses its focus on unpleasant events. A pleasant "high" is achieved with strenuous and protracted exercise. After exercise, you feel tired and refreshed at the same time, due to the brain's release of endorphins, which are mood-elevating chemicals associated with a sense of well-being. Phenylethylamine, another chemical associated with energy and a happier mood, also increases with exercise. Not to mention that weight loss is easier and muscle mass increases, improving your appearance. The bottom line is that you become buff, de-stressed, and happier. Try to do all that with a pill!

Get Sufficient Sleep

Even with our activity-filled, busy days at the Pritikin Center, we stress the importance of getting a good night's sleep. Chronic sleep deprivation is a major cause of accidents, impaired productivity, and disease. It may be difficult to sleep well during a period of acute stress, but sleep is a great antidote to chronic stress.

Almost as many Americans have trouble sleeping as are overweight.

Unfortunately, they also understand good sleeping habits about as much as they understand a good diet. Here are some ways to improve your quality—and quantity—of sleep:

- Exercise regularly to burn off accumulated stress, but avoid exercising in the evening.
- Do not nap during the day and avoid stimulants in the evening, such as caffeine.
- Do not eat big meals or drink alcohol within three or four hours of bedtime. Both may make you initially sleepy, but they disturb refreshing sleep.
- Lose weight if you need to. Obesity is associated with irregular breathing, termed obstructive sleep apnea, which interferes with sleep. Snoring and waking up frequently may also be signs of obstructive sleep apnea.
- Sleep in a quiet, dark, and comfortable room.
- Go to sleep at a regular bedtime. Although we differ in the amount of sleep we individually need, seven hours is a reasonable average.
- If you are not getting enough sleep because you have kids, adjust your schedule to more closely model your kids' so that you can sleep when they sleep.
- If you don't fall asleep within 20 or 30 minutes, do not remain awake in bed. Get up and read or do something else until you feel sleepy.
- Do not work in bed. Reserve your bed for sleep.
- If you develop chronic insomnia, get medical help. It may be the first symptom of depression or some other emotional disturbance.

Develop Close Relationships

Social connectedness is important for physical and emotional health. Meaningful social relationships lead to successful aging as much as a healthy lifestyle does.

Most people already know how talking with a friend reduces stress and increases happiness. As much as you can—or as much as you personally feel you need—spend time with friends with at least some similar interests and core values. That advice applies especially to marriage, which is the ultimate social connectedness. Married people, by the way, do live longer than singles, especially if they are happily married. Yet another good reason to be emotionally nourishing to and with your spouse!

Laugh

Humor is one of the best antidotes for stress. The physical activity of laughing relaxes our muscles, and can turn even the most troubling circumstance into a relaxing one. As we already mentioned, humorous entertainment has real physical benefit.

As often as you can, try to find the humor in life. The rewards are both immediate and long-term. Besides, who doesn't love a good laugh?

Have Physical Contact

Being touched by others is an essential human need. Babies who are not held do not develop and grow as they should. In a sense, we do not change as we become adults. Touch relaxes and bonds people in a way that no conversation can. From hand holding to cuddling and caressing, touch creates an intense sense of well-being in most people.

The ultimate touch—sexual activity—is more than a means of reproduction. Sexual activity releases stress and can mend even the bitterest argument with a partner or spouse. Touch and sexual relations stimulate the brain to release the hormone oxytocin, which is one of the hormones that bind people together (it is also associated with nursing). Oxytocin speeds wound healing and may decrease the risk of some cancers. Endorphins are also released during sex, as with exercise.

Sexual activity burns 100 to 200 calories, or the equivalent of walking one to two miles. Now, I know what you are thinking: "Do I have to walk if I have an active sex life?" The answer is yes. We want you to enjoy both long walks *and* committed and responsible sexual activities!

Sex and Your Heart

Does sexual activity reduce heart disease? Studies say yes. In one 10-year study, men who had sex two or more times per week experienced half as many heart attacks as did those who had sex less than once per month. In another study, college students who engaged in sexual activity once or twice per week had higher immunity to infection than those who abstained.

Get Canine Companions

Get a dog and walk it. Better yet, get a few dogs! It's been shown that pet owners are much more likely to survive a heart attack, especially if they have one or more dogs. Some studies have found that dogs protect against heart disease more than cats. Now, I know that there are wonderful cats out there; in fact, my wife and I have had several very sociable feline companions. But dogs foster a better lifestyle. People walk dogs, or better said, dogs walk people. In addition to the physical activity, walking around your neighborhood introduces you to new neighbors, especially if they are also dog walkers, and social connectivity is, as we know, good for the heart.

Dog owners have less heart disease even when the added walking is factored out. Why are dogs so wonderful for our health? They are the quintessential stress-reducing, emotionally nourishing beings. Think about it: you can feel stress evaporate by petting a dog. The effect is very real; several studies have shown that blood pressure and pulse decrease with petting. Dogs are happy, loving creatures whose natural love of life is infectious, and who couldn't benefit from that?

Make Time for Enjoyable Activities

We Americans work more hours than anyone else in the world. As a consequence of overworking, we have surrendered our diet to the fast-food industry, given up on exercise, and relinquished time for personal enjoyment. Heart disease, diabetes, obesity, insomnia, depression, and shorter life span are the direct consequences. Are bigger houses and faster cars worth this high price? We must think so, because we are not slowing down. If we don't, however, nature and heart disease will do it for us.

Take time in your life for family, friends, hobbies, and vacations. They are the reasons why we work. The positive action of taking time for ourselves puts us in control of our own lives, which in turn reduces stress.

Vacations recharge our internal batteries. American executives sometimes brag that it has been years since they took a real vacation. In a nine-year study, people who didn't take annual vacations were 21 percent more likely to die and 32 percent more likely to die of heart disease. Take vacations. When we say vacations, we mean *relaxing* vacations; it is not necessary to visit 19 cities in two days! And, as a side note, we feel compelled to add: don't use a vacation as an excuse to overeat. The 15 pounds you gain will undo the benefits of relaxation.

Develop Spiritually

One healthy characteristic of the American lifestyle is widespread spirituality and religious belief. Spirituality is a belief in a higher power and meaning of life. It gives life purpose. Religion—the organization of spirituality into practice—generally teaches the values of healthy lifestyle, marriage, family, community, education, and work. Religions discourage the excesses of overeating, inactivity, smoking, and alcohol abuse. Spirituality and religion reduce stress because they provide hope and a sense of control. After all, prayer beats worry.

More than half of middle-aged and elderly Americans use religious faith as a coping mechanism when ill. Their faith is not unfounded: people who regularly attend religious services live eight years longer than people who don't.

One of the best ways to nourish yourself spiritually is to do something good for someone else. Volunteering changes your focus from your own troubled thoughts to helping others. If you like exercise, try coaching a children's sports team. If you like to talk, tutor. If you want to change our culture, get involved in politics. Helping others helps you as much as it helps them.

Meditation, Tai Chi, and Yoga

Meditation, tai chi, and yoga are the "medications" of relaxation. Learning these ancient Eastern techniques fully requires more instruction than we can provide in this book, but there are many terrific classes available that you can join to learn more. At Pritikin, there's nothing more fun than watching guests who came in thinking that "yoga is for weirdoes," including some of the Fortune 500 CEOs. Often, they're the very same guys who end up swearing that yoga—the soft music, gentle movements, and soothing voice of our yoga instructor—is even better than nap time in kindergarten.

Meditation is designed to focus your mind and bring it into the present. It also happens to lower pulse and blood pressure. Meditation focuses your thoughts on a repeated word or your breathing to calm anxieties. Try this simple exercise: Find a quiet place and sit in a relaxed posture. Slowly repeat a simple, pleasant-sounding word that ends gradually, such as "stream." Alternatively, you can focus on your quiet breathing, using your abdominal muscles rather than just your chest. If distracting thoughts come into your head, accept them without judgment and let them go. Continue your focus on the world or your breathing for 15 to 20 minutes. You will feel yourself relax.

Tai chi is a form of physical meditation that involves slow, flowing, disciplined movements. Those who wish to be more physically active might prefer it to meditation.

Yoga involves body postures, slow breathing, and rest. The postures, held for several breaths, strengthen muscles and increase flexibility.

We Americans may lead the world in work and productivity, but other cultures are more advanced at relaxation. We could certainly stand to learn a thing or two from them.

KEY POINTS TO REMEMBER

- Stress is not created by our circumstances; it is created by how we respond to our circumstances.
- Stress contributes to heart disease.
- To reduce stress:
  —Become emotionally nourishing.
  —Exercise regularly.
  —Get sufficient sleep.
  —Develop close relationships.
  —Laugh.
  —Touch others and enjoy a regular sexual relationship.
  —Get a pet, especially a dog.
  —Reserve time for enjoyable activities.
  —Develop spiritually.
  —Consider meditation, tai chi, and/or yoga.

15

If at First You Don't Succeed . . .

THERE'S A WONDERFUL Japanese proverb that says, "Fall down seven times, stand up eight." I want you to keep this proverb in mind as you launch your healthier life. Remember, everyone makes mistakes. *Everyone.* But mistakes do not mean failure. The only time you fail is when you stop trying. The eighth, nine, or tenth time that you pull yourself up may be the time that you *stay up.* It worked for Joe, a recurring Pritikin guest who kept at it until he got it right. Read on.

CASE STUDY: JOE

Joe, 62 years old and a retired civil engineer, was never chubby or a couch potato in his youth. A lover of the outdoors, he scaled mountains, hiked the California deserts, volunteered at cheetah conservation preserves in Africa, and in 1973 became a Sierra Club hike leader.

In his late 40s, Joe started putting on weight, ballooning up to 240 pounds and beyond. "Not much leading of Sierra hikes was going on at that time," he recalls. Fed up with being fat, he came to the Pritikin Longevity Center in 1998, his first of several visits over the next seven years. His weight plunged 70 pounds following that first visit, but maintaining the weight loss was a different ball game.

Between 1998 and 2005, Joe regained the weight between visits to Pritikin. Then he suffered a nasty fall from a slick log on a mountain trail that left him more hobbler than hiker, and he gained more weight. "I was just drinking too much, eating too much, and not moving enough," he admits.

Finally, in March 2005, Joe booked a flight to Pritikin and resolved, "I've really got to *do it* this time. I'm 272 pounds."

This time, it clicked. Joe dropped 115 pounds and has kept it off for the last three years. He's now a slim, Sierra-ready 157 pounds. Every single day he works up a sweat, either at the YMCA or hiking in the local mountains.

His secret to success "started not in the body, but in the brain," he says. "The body will do what it's told. If the brain is not in gear, it's not going to work. That's what I've learned these past few years. I'd be a billionaire if I could just tell people how to turn that brain switch 'on.' But I can't. I'm not sure why it happened."

What Joe does know is that he banished the thought that he was deprived. "As long as you think you're losing something, you're going to want it back. For me, Pritikin is not about deprivation. Pritikin is about *enjoying good healthy food.* Another 'D' word I've banished is 'diet.' I'm not dieting. I'm just *eating well.*"

Eating well is no longer a chore. Joe loves buffets, especially in restaurants like Sizzler and Souplantation. "Oh, sure," he says, "you can kill yourself at a buffet, but you can save yourself, too. I always head straight for the salad bars and fill up a plate—a *big* plate—with spinach and other veggies. Then I go back and get something else, usually more vegetables!"

He does the same thing when traveling. "My wife and I were in Turkey recently, eating a lot at nice hotel buffets. For breakfast, I'd fill two or three bowls with cherries. People were amazed. At dinner, I'd start out with a huge plate of vegetables, avoid the cheeses and other greasy foods, order broiled or steamed fish, and finish with a big bowl of fruit for dessert."

Last but not least, Joe knocked off the beer. About two and a half years ago, he went to an ear, nose, and throat specialist because his throat was bothering him. The doctor very pointedly told him that alcohol was causing a real problem, acid reflux. He needed to give it up. Joe did, and "it was the best thing for my weight-loss efforts because beer has *so many calories.* I was drinking a six-pack a day. Well, if I say I'm on the Pritikin Program with the exception of a six-pack a day, that's one hell of an exception. Once I stopped taking in several hundred liquid calories every day, losing weight and keeping it off got much easier.

"Have I given beer up completely? No. I just save it for special occasions. Planning for Turkey, I told myself that I wasn't going to turn down local brews, so I allowed myself one a day. It's not that hard to drink zero beers. It's damn hard to drink one. It was a test, and thankfully I passed it. I was able to drink one Turkish beer. Some days, in fact, I didn't drink any at all."

It's all worth it, Joe affirms, because he gets to live precisely the type of life he wants to live in his retirement years. "There's a lot to enjoy these days! Great health, loads of energy, hiking in Griffith Park with my wife and friends on Wednesday nights, going to the local mountains in fall, winter, and spring. I've got my life back! And I feel fantastic—*every* day."

Let's review the essentials of how Joe lost 115 pounds and kept it off.

- Commitment to a real lifestyle change
- Lots of fruits, vegetables, and fish
- Elimination of high-calorie beverages
- Daily enjoyable physical activity

Like Joe, you may have tried before. Well, try it again with a better plan. This time it just might stick.

MARGARET'S THIRD VISIT

Margaret came back, again with a smile on her face. She had lost 14 pounds total in three months, as much as I wanted her to lose by then. Though she was delighted with her success thus far, she confided in me that she had lost 15 pounds several times before in less time, only to have them quickly return. I reminded her that this was exactly why we were aiming to lose the weight slowly, through enjoyable lifestyle changes, so that this time, as with Joe, it would stick. Margaret nodded and said she was optimistic because she didn't feel that she was on a diet.

Moreover, life was good. She liked the food she was now eating better, and certainly wasn't hungry. Her dog had even lost two pounds, and she and her husband were getting along terrifically. She had already dropped two dress sizes and had bought a few new outfits, one of which was a bathing suit that she would use for an upcoming trip to Mexico her husband had signed them up for, perhaps, Margaret laughed, because he wanted to see her in said bathing suit! Her coworkers were supportive, complimenting her often about how much thinner and healthier she looked. Her new weight and life-style was doing her good, and it showed.

I asked Margaret what she was doing for exercise, and she excitedly told me that in addition to her daily walks with her husband and dog, she had revived her love of tennis (she played in high school) and joined a women's tennis league that played for two hours twice a week at their community facility. She wore her pedometer when she played and was delighted to see that she was well over 10,000 steps on those days. Margaret was amazed to find that she was still competitive, even with younger players. Besides the league play, she had accepted several invitations to play other matches, and had already signed up for another indoor winter league. She had a lovely, healthy glow to her skin, and had obviously crossed over from couch potato to fitness fan.

The best news of all was Margaret's blood pressure and cholesterol pro-file. Her blood pressure on this visit was 130 over 80, a full eight points lower than when she first visited me. Her LDL (bad) cholesterol had fallen from 130 to 108 and her HDL (good) cholesterol was up from 50 to 55. Her lower blood pressure had reduced her heart disease risk by 30 percent; her lower LDL (bad) cholesterol had reduced her risk by 30 percent, and her increase in HDL (good) cholesterol had reduced it by 20 percent. In just three months, she had decreased her overall risk of having a heart attack by *more than 60 percent*.

I knew that Margaret's weight loss and low-salt diet played big roles in her improved blood pressure and cholesterol, but I was interested in what other changes she had made. Margaret had switched margarines to a stanol-containing brand (see Chapter 11) and was using two pats daily. She and her husband were surprised that it tasted much like the margarine they had been eating. She cooked with either that or canola oil.

Speaking of cooking, Margaret was eating more fish, and had gotten into the habit of asking the fishmonger at the supermarket about which fish were really fresh and for a few preparation suggestions. She had also discovered that her upscale supermarket had fresh fish already marinated and ready to cook. She'd thrown out all the salt at home and was experimenting more with healthier seasonings. She'd become not only a fitness fan, but a fan of food. No longer did she view food as the enemy.

Margaret was gaining control of her diet, weight, and health—and hence, her happiness. She liked the feeling, especially when her husband raved about her meals. I told Margaret to come back in a year or when she got down to 132 pounds, our goal, whichever came first.

PART THREE

Favorite Pritikin Recipes

HERE IS A collection of our favorite recipes and tips for foods for all occasions and times of the day. Dive right in! They're the creations of the talented chefs at Pritikin. These recipes have met the toughest test of all: the approval of the guests at the Pritikin Longevity Center, many of whom are accustomed to eating at the finest restaurants in the world. The chefs at Pritikin aim to duplicate that experience as much as possible, and present food that's not only healthy but absolutely delicious.

The job of the doctors and dietitians at Pritikin is to teach people *why* they want to follow the Pritikin Program, and the chefs show them how doable it is. The compliment they cherish most is when guests say, "I like what I'm eating so much that I *know* I can do this at home. Thank you!"

Note: All of the following salad dressings and sauces should be stored in the refrigerator in airtight containers and will last up to a week.

Enjoy your time in the kitchen—and the good health and weight loss that will follow.

Salad Dressings

Let's start with salad dressings, because they can make or break both the healthiness and waist-popping potential of any salad. Pour gobs of fat-laden dressing on a salad and you might as well be eating a cheeseburger. When dining out, ask your server to leave off the regular dressing (which probably adds 400 to 600 calories to your salad). Here are some delicious alternatives, all much lower in calories (about five to 25 calories per two-tablespoon serving). In most cases, they're lower in sodium, too.

Vinegars: Ask for traditional varieties like balsamic and red wine vinegars or more exotic options like champagne vinegar and muscat grape vinegar. Simply ask your server, "What's in the kitchen? What types of vinegars is the chef using?" Then request that a bottle be brought out for your salad. Be sure to read the label, as some chefs use salted vinegars. Rice vinegar, for example, is often salted.

Lemon Juice: At home, squeeze fresh lemon juice on cut pieces of apple and avocado to keep them from turning brown. In a restaurant, ask for lemon juice to add zest to many vegetables. It may even suffice as a salad dressing when you're really trying to lose weight.

Fresh Salsa: Again, find out what's in the kitchen. Sometimes there may be exotic salsas the chef has whipped up as a topping for seafood, like a fresh papaya and cilantro salsa, which would make a fabulous dressing for your salad.

Wasabi and Rice Vinegar: In Asian-style restaurants, add a lot of kick to your salads by adding a bit of wasabi (known as Japanese horseradish) to rice vinegar. Want it hotter? Add more wasabi. Stir and pour.

Shrimp-Cocktail-Style Dressing: If the menu has shrimp cocktail sauce, ask for some on the side with your salad. If it is not on the menu, make your own. Ask for ketchup and a little horseradish, and a little dish to stir up the two ingredients.

Low-Calorie Vinaigrette: Ask for a cruet of olive, canola, or walnut oil and one of vinegar. Pour mostly vinegar with just a teaspoon or less of oil. Season with black pepper.

Dijon and Balsamic: Request a bottle of Dijon mustard and one of balsamic vinegar. Pour some of each in a small dish, stir it up, and pour over your salad

Zesty and Creamy: Health-conscious restaurants may have fat-free sour cream or yogurt in the kitchen. If so, ask for an ounce or two and sass it up with mustard, balsamic vinegar, ketchup, or hot sauce.

Banana and Rice Wine Vinaigrette

MAKES ABOUT 4 CUPS

1 very ripe banana

1 teaspoon minced garlic

1 tablespoon chopped fresh cilantro leaves

¼ cup cucumber, diced small

2 cups rice vinegar

1 cup water

3 tablespoons chili paste

In a large bowl, mash the banana with a whisk. Add remaining ingredients. Whip by hand until well combined.

Note: All dressings will last in the fridge for about one week, and yes, store in a covered container.

Note: This Banana/Rice Wine dressing will change color, so it's best to use it within 2 to 3 days.

Nutrition Information (per 2-tablespoon serving): 4 calories, 0g fat, 0g saturated fat, 0mg cholesterol, less than 1g protein, less than 1g fiber, less than 1mg sodium.

Basil Cucumber Vinaigrette

MAKES ABOUT 4 CUPS

3 cucumbers, peeled, seeded,* and chopped to fit in a blender

½ cup fresh basil leaves

¼ cup fresh lemon juice

½ teaspoon black peppercorns, ground

4 tablespoons Z Trim**

½ cup white vinegar

In a blender, blend all ingredients until smooth.

Nutrition Information (per 2-tablespoon serving): 3 calories, 0g fat, 0g saturated fat, 0mg cholesterol, less than 1g protein, less than 1g fiber, 4mg sodium.

————

* To seed a cucumber, peel and cut in half lengthwise. With a teaspoon, scoop out seeds and discard.

** Z Trim is a zero-calorie fat replacement gel made from corn developed at the Agricultural Research Service of the U.S. Department of Agriculture. Currently it is available online at www.ztrim.com.

Champagne Vinaigrette

MAKES 3 TO 4 CUPS

1 cup champagne vinegar

1 cup Z Trim (see page 181 for information on obtaining Z Trim)

2 tablespoons low-sodium Dijon mustard

1 shallot, minced

1 garlic clove, minced

¼ cup minced chives

1 cucumber, peeled, seeded, and minced

1 red bell pepper, minced

In a large bowl, mix all ingredients with a whisk until well combined.

Nutrition Information (per 2-tablespoon serving): 3 calories, 0g fat, 0g saturated fat, 0mg cholesterol, less than 1g protein, less than 1g fiber, 25mg sodium.

Creamy-Style House Dressing

MAKES ABOUT 3 CUPS

¾ cup plain fat-free yogurt

½ cup fat-free sour cream

¾ cup low-sodium, fruit-sweetened ketchup (such as Westbrae brand)

½ teaspoon dry oregano

½ teaspoon granulated garlic

½ cup nonfat milk

In a large bowl, mix all ingredients until well combined.

Nutrition Information (per 2-tablespoon serving): 17 calories, 0g fat, 0g saturated fat, less than 1mg cholesterol, less than 1g protein, 0g fiber, 16mg sodium.

Cucumber Yogurt Dill Dressing

This is a very versatile recipe. It's fabulous not only as a salad dressing but also as a sauce for chicken and seafood, particularly salmon, and as a topping for baked potatoes.

MAKES ABOUT 4 CUPS

3 English (hothouse) cucumbers, peeled and chopped

¼ cup white balsamic vinegar

¼ cup fresh lime or lemon juice

¼ bunch fresh dill, chopped

2 cups fat-free plain yogurt

½ cup fat-free sour cream

In a food processor, purée the cucumbers with the vinegar until smooth and thick. Pour in a large mixing bowl. Add remaining ingredients, and mix with a whisk until well combined. Chill and serve.

Nutrition Information (per 2-tablespoon serving): 10 calories, less than 1g fat, 0g saturated fat, less than 1mg cholesterol, less than 1g protein, 0g fiber, 9mg sodium.

Honey Mustard Dressing

MAKES ABOUT 3 CUPS

6 ounces Westbrae Stoneground Mustard, No Salt

1 ounce Westbrae Dijon style mustard

4 tablespoons white vinegar

4 tablespoons water

½ teaspoon finely chopped garlic

1 teaspoon dried oregano

2 tablespoons frozen apple juice concentrate

1 cup fat-free sour cream

In a blender, blend all ingredients until creamy.

Nutrition Information (per 2-tablespoon serving): 11 calories, less than 1g fat, 0g saturated fat, 1mg cholesterol, less than 1g protein, 0g fiber, 34mg sodium.

Horseradish-Balsamic Vinaigrette

MAKES ABOUT 1½ CUPS

2 tablespoons horseradish

1 cup balsamic vinegar

2 teaspoons low-sodium Dijon mustard

1 teaspoon frozen apple juice concentrate

In a medium-size bowl, mix all ingredients with a whisk until well combined.

Nutrition Information (per 2-tablespoon serving): 18 calories, 0g fat, 0g saturated fat, 0mg cholesterol, 0g protein, less than 1g fiber, 29mg sodium.

Raita

Raita is a South Asian yogurt-based condiment used as a sauce or dip as well as a salad dressing. It pairs well with greens, seafood, raw veggie appetizers like celery and radishes, and can be used as a sauce over lentils or brown rice.

MAKES ABOUT 3 CUPS

1 medium tomato, diced

1 ½ cups plain nonfat yogurt

2 tablespoons fresh, finely chopped mint leaves

¼ cup finely chopped scallions or mild onion

1 small cucumber, peeled, seeded, and diced

½ tablespoon toasted and ground cumin seeds*

Pepper and Tabasco, to taste

In a large bowl, combine all ingredients. Chill at least 30 minutes before serving.

Nutrition Information (per ½-cup serving): 36 calories, less than 1g fat, 0g saturated fat, 1mg cholesterol, 3g protein, less than 1g fiber, 37mg sodium.

---

* To toast cumin, place seeds over high heat in a small heavy skillet on the stove. Toss them frequently until fragrant, about 2 to 4 minutes.

Raspberry Vinaigrette

MAKES ABOUT 2 ½ CUPS

1 cup fresh raspberries (If fresh berries are not available, use frozen no-sugar-added
  berries.)
1 cup fresh blackberries
½ cup white balsamic vinegar
½ bunch of fresh dill, chopped
1 tablespoon Splenda, or to taste
½ teaspoon black peppercorns, ground

In a blender, blend all ingredients until smooth. Adjust taste and consistency with water, additional vinegar, and/or Splenda, depending on size and sweetness of berries.

Nutrition Information (per 2-tablespoon serving): 12 calories, 0g fat, 0g saturated fat, 0mg cholesterol, less than 1g protein, 1g fiber, 3mg sodium.

Sauces

Homemade sauces are especially helpful if you're trying to cut down on sodium. A typical serving of store-bought barbecue sauce, for example, has about 500 milligrams of sodium, whereas our recipe on the next page has only 16 milligrams.

Note: All sauces will last in the fridge for about one week, stored in a covered container.

Barbecue Sauce

MAKES ABOUT 2½ CUPS

1 tablespoon peeled and minced ginger

¼ cup minced garlic

1 jalapeño pepper, seeded and diced

2 ounces frozen apple juice concentrate

½ cup apple cider vinegar

2 ounces no-salt-added stone-ground mustard (such as Westbrae brand)

1 tablespoon low-sodium Dijon mustard

1 ½ pounds low-sodium tomato puree

½ teaspoon black peppercorns, ground

1 teaspoon dry oregano

½ teaspoon liquid smoke

In a large stockpot, cook the ginger, garlic, jalapeño, apple juice, and vinegar over medium heat, stirring occasionally. Reduce until the consistency of syrup, about 12 minutes. Add remaining ingredients and mix until well combined. Raise heat and bring to a boil. Reduce heat, and simmer for 1 hour. Use immediately, or store in an airtight container in the refrigerator for up to 1 week.

Nutrition Information (per 3-tablespoon serving): 22 calories, 0g fat, 0g saturated fat, 0mg cholesterol, less than 1g protein, 1g fiber, 16mg sodium.

Creamy Dill Sauce

This is a rich and tangy sauce for poultry as well as poached or baked seafood.

MAKES ABOUT 3 CUPS

2 tablespoons chopped garlic

2 tablespoons chopped shallots

1 cup dry white wine

2 bay leaves

12 ounces silken tofu

2 tablespoons fat-free sour cream

3 tablespoons apple cider vinegar

2 ounces water

1 tablespoon low-sodium Dijon mustard

3 tablespoons chopped fresh dill

In a hot nonstick saucepan, brown the garlic and shallots. Deglaze with the wine to loosen and dissolve brown bits at the bottom of the pan. Add the bay leaves and reduce mixture by half. In a large bowl, blend the tofu, sour cream, vinegar, water, and mustard until smooth. Add tofu mixture to reduction, and simmer over low heat until sauce is thickened. Remove the bay leaves, add the chopped dill, and serve.

Nutrition Information (per 2-tablespoon serving): 19 calories, less than 1g fat, 0g saturated fat, less than 1mg cholesterol, 1g protein, 0g fiber, 7mg sodium.

Curry Sauce

This is a versatile sauce. You can use it with everything from vegetables and tofu to chicken and fish. Plus, it freezes well.

MAKES ABOUT 3 CUPS

½ pound chopped onion

1 tablespoon chopped garlic

¼ pound chopped tomatoes

1 teaspoon ground ginger

1 teaspoon ground cumin

1 teaspoon ground coriander

½ teaspoon freshly ground allspice

1 tablespoon chopped fresh thyme leaves

1 teaspoon madras curry powder

½ teaspoon turmeric

2 cups water

½ teaspoon cayenne pepper

1 tablespoon chopped cilantro leaves (optional)

2 tablespoons chopped scallion greens (the tips of the scallions)

In a hot nonstick skillet, sauté the onion, garlic, tomatoes, and ginger until softened. Add the cumin, coriander, allspice, thyme, curry powder, and turmeric. Cook for 3 minutes more. Add the water and cook over low heat for 20 minutes. Add the cayenne and cilantro, if using. Just before serving, add the scallions.

Nutrition Information (per 1-cup serving): 11 calories, less than 1g fat, 0g saturated fat, 0mg cholesterol, less than 1g protein, less than 1g fiber, 2mg sodium.

Fresh Tomato Sauce

MAKES ABOUT 4 CUPS

8 large tomatoes

¼ cup diced onion

¼ cup chopped garlic

½ teaspoon dried oregano

¼ teaspoon black peppercorns, ground

½ teaspoon dried basil

1 teaspoon Splenda

¼ bunch fresh basil leaves, sliced into very thin strips

Cut, grate, or purée the tomatoes, as desired. In a nonstick saucepan over medium heat, brown the onions and garlic. Add the tomatoes, oregano, and pepper. Cook over medium heat until thickened, about 40 minutes. Mix in the Splenda and fresh basil.

Nutrition Information (per 1-cup serving): 86 calories, less than 1g total fat, less than 1g saturated fat, 0mg cholesterol, 4g protein, 5g fiber, 20mg sodium.

Jerk Seasoning

This is a very spicy marinade, fantastic with seafood, poultry, and vegetables.

MAKES 3 CUPS

1 pound scallions

1 pound Vidalia onions

3 Scotch bonnet chili peppers or 3 habañero chili peppers

1 teaspoon freshly ground allspice

¼ cup chopped garlic

2 tablespoons chopped fresh thyme leaves

1 tablespoon grated fresh ginger

1 teaspoon low-sodium soy sauce

¼ cup low-sodium vegetable stock (such as Pritikin recipe)

¼ cup balsamic vinegar

Rough-chop the scallions, onions, and peppers. Combine all ingredients and blend in a food processor for 5 minutes. Let marinate in refrigerator overnight before using.

Nutrition Information (per 2-tablespoon serving): 11 calories, 0g fat, 0g saturated fat, 0mg cholesterol, less than 1g protein, less than 1g fiber, 7mg sodium.

Pico de Gallo

MAKES 2 CUPS

2 large tomatoes, diced

½ red onion, finely chopped

½ jalapeño pepper, very finely chopped (remove seeds for a milder salsa)

2 tablespoons chopped cilantro leaves

2 limes, juiced

Pinch black peppercorns, ground

In a medium bowl, mix all ingredients and let sit for 15 minutes before serving.

Nutrition Information (per ½ cup serving): 20 calories, less than 1g fat, 0g saturated fat, 0mg cholesterol, less than 1g protein, 1g fiber, 4mg sodium.

Tofu Mayonnaise

MAKES 4 CUPS

Three 12-ounce boxes of silken tofu

1 ½ tablespoons low-sodium Dijon mustard

3 tablespoons white balsamic vinegar

1 teaspoon low-sodium Worcestershire sauce

1 dash Tabasco

1 teaspoon minced garlic

1 teaspoon finely chopped shallots

In a large bowl, combine all ingredients. Refrigerate.

Nutrition Information (per 1-tablespoon serving): 7 calories, less than 1g fat, 0g saturated fat, 0mg cholesterol, 1g protein, 0g fiber, 21mg sodium.

Soups

Soups, as you know, are a mainstay of the Pritikin diet. Any of the following will make for a wonderful, filling start to your meals—or a meal by itself.

All soups freeze well. Our recipes make larger quantities to save and freeze so they can be enjoyed in a variety of ways every day, from snacks to meals.

Black Bean Soup

MAKES 8 CUPS

2 cups dry black beans, soaked overnight, rinsed, and drained

2 red onions, diced

½ cup chopped garlic

1 tablespoon cumin, ground fresh

2 teaspoons coriander, ground fresh

1 teaspoon oregano

1 chipotle pepper (whole)

1 carrot, diced

½ teaspoon black peppercorns, ground

3 quarts water

¼ to ½ cup chopped cilantro leaves

In a large stockpot over medium heat, simmer all ingredients, except cilantro, stirring occasionally until the beans are soft, about 2 to 3 hours. When ready to serve, remove the chipotle pepper and add the cilantro.

Nutrition Information (per 1-cup serving): 164 calories, less than 1g fat, less than 1g saturated fat, 0mg cholesterol, 10g protein, 7g fiber, 16mg sodium.

Butternut Squash Soup

MAKES 8 CUPS

1 cup chopped onions

1 butternut squash, peeled and chopped

2 tablespoons minced garlic

1 teaspoon low-sodium soy sauce

½ teaspoon white pepper

2 tablespoons frozen apple juice concentrate

2 quarts low-sodium vegetable stock (such as Pritikin recipe)

1 cup minced Italian parsley

1 tablespoon fresh thyme, leaves picked from stems

Preheat oven to 400°F.

Place the chopped onions and half of the squash on a nonstick baking tray and roast in oven until fork tender, about 25 minutes. In a food processor purée the onions and squash. Add purée and remaining ingredients, except the parsley and thyme, to a stockpot. Adjust seasonings to taste, if needed. Cook on stove over medium heat for about 20 minutes. Stir in the parsley and thyme.

Nutrition Information (per 1-cup serving): 116 calories, less than 1g fat, 0g saturated fat, 0mg cholesterol, 3g protein, 6g fiber, 66mg sodium.

Corn Chowder

MAKES 10 CUPS

1 carrot, chopped

½ cup peeled, chopped potatoes

1½ cups chopped onions

¼ cup minced garlic

¼ pound okra

2 stalks celery, chopped

1 quart low-sodium vegetable broth (such as Pritikin recipe)

½ tablespoon dried oregano

½ teaspoon celery seed

2 teaspoons cumin seeds, ground

½ teaspoon black pepper

1 bay leaf

1 cup nonfat milk

1 teaspoon low-sodium soy sauce

1 pound frozen corn, thawed

1 teaspoon chopped Italian parsley leaves

Steam the carrots until tender and set aside.

In a large saucepan, sauté the potatoes, onions, garlic, okra, and celery in one-third of the vegetable broth for 10 minutes. Add the remaining broth and spices, bring to a boil, and simmer for 30 minutes. Remove the bay leaf and add the milk and soy sauce. Purée the soup using either a food processor or handheld blender. Add the corn and carrots. Return to the pan and simmer for 15 minutes more. Garnish with the chopped parsley.

Nutrition Information (per 1-cup serving): 96 calories, less than 1g fat, less than 1g saturated fat, less than 1mg cholesterol, 4g protein, 4g fiber, 64mg sodium.

Eight Bean Soup

MAKES 16 CUPS

1 pound of assorted dry beans, such as split peas, yellow split peas, lentils, red, black,
  pigeon, navy, kidney, white, or lima beans, green lentils, and crimson lentils
1 yellow bell pepper, diced
1 green bell pepper, diced
1 red bell pepper, diced
¼ cup chopped garlic
¼ cup chopped shallots
1 red onion, diced
2 quarts water
1 tablespoon dried oregano
1 teaspoon chili powder
1 teaspoon liquid smoke
1 teaspoon garlic powder
8 ounces no-salt-added salsa (such as Enrico's)
¼ cup balsamic vinegar
1 pint Knudsen Very Veggie Juice, low sodium
¼ bunch cilantro, leaves picked and chopped

Soak beans overnight, rinse, and drain.

In a large stockpot, cook the bell peppers, garlic, shallots, and onion
until soft. Add the beans, water, oregano, chili powder, liquid smoke,
garlic powder, salsa, vinegar, and juice. Stir and simmer for 2½ hours.
When ready to serve, garnish with the cilantro.

Nutrition Information (per 1-cup serving): 123 calories, less than 1g fat, less than
1g saturated fat, 0mg cholesterol, 7g protein, 5g fiber, 34mg sodium.

Garbanzo and Spinach Soup

MAKES 9 CUPS

2 tablespoons minced garlic

1 onion, diced

2 teaspoons ground cumin

2 teaspoons ground coriander

½ teaspoon cayenne pepper

½ teaspoon black peppercorns, ground

1 quart low-sodium vegetable stock (such as Pritikin recipe)

3 potatoes, peeled and diced

One 14.5-ounce can of no-salt-added chickpeas (garbanzo beans)

1 cup nonfat milk

1 tablespoon tahini paste

1 tablespoon cornstarch

2 cups sliced spinach leaves

In a large nonstick saucepan, sauté the garlic and onion until light brown. Add the spices, vegetable stock, and potatoes, and cook over medium heat for 15 minutes. Add the chickpeas, and cook for 5 minutes more.

In a medium-sized bowl, mix together the milk, tahini, and cornstarch. Add to soup mixture. Add spinach, and cook for 2 minutes more.

Nutrition Information (per 1-cup serving): 129 calories, 1½ g fat, less than 1g saturated fat, 0mg cholesterol, 8g protein, 5g fiber, 79mg sodium.

Green Chile and Tomato Soup

MAKES 14 CUPS

3 cups canned diced tomatoes, no-salt-added

2 onions, peeled and sliced

1 potato, peeled and diced

1 carrot, peeled and sliced

2 tablespoons chopped fresh thyme leaves

4 tablespoons minced garlic

1 tablespoon cumin seeds, toasted and ground (see page 185)

1 tablespoon paprika

1 cup canned diced green chilies

2 quarts low-sodium vegetable stock (such as Pritikin recipe)

2 scallions, sliced

2 tablespoons chopped fresh cilantro leaves

In a stockpot, add all ingredients except the scallions and cilantro. Cook over medium heat, stirring occasionally, until all ingredients are soft, about 1 hour. Add the scallions and cilantro. Cook for 3 minutes more.

Nutrition Information (per 1-cup serving): 45 calories, less than 1g fat, 0g saturated fat, 0mg cholesterol, 2g protein, 3g fiber, 32mg sodium.

Mushroom and Edamame Soup

Edamame is the Japanese name for fresh soybeans. They're often available in the frozen section of markets.

MAKES 12 CUPS

1 cup uncooked edamame

1 onion, peeled and sliced

2 cups quartered domestic mushrooms

2 cups sliced shiitake mushrooms

1 carrot, peeled and sliced

2 tablespoons chopped lemongrass*

2 tablespoons minced garlic

1 tablespoon ginger powder

1 teaspoon wasabi powder

1 tablespoon chopped fresh ginger

2 quarts water

1 cup sliced snow peas

2 tablespoons chopped fresh cilantro leaves

2 scallions, sliced

In a stockpot, add all ingredients except the snow peas, cilantro, and scallions. Cook over medium heat, stirring occasionally, until all ingredients are just soft, about 20 minutes. Add the snow peas, cilantro, and scallions. Cook for 2 minutes more.

Nutrition Information (per 1-cup serving): 46 calories, less than 1g fat, less than 1g saturated fat, 0mg cholesterol, 3g protein, 2g fiber, 20mg sodium.

---

* Use the bulb's soft interior only. To get to the bulb of each lemongrass stalk, beat the stalk with the back of a knife and peel away until you get to the soft interior. Each stalk yields about 1 teaspoon.

Spiced Lentil Soup

MAKES 16 CUPS

1 pound red lentils

2 onions, chopped

4 cloves garlic, minced

4 stalks celery, sliced

½ teaspoon kosher salt

1 teaspoon black peppercorns, ground

1 teaspoon turmeric

1 teaspoon cumin

¼ teaspoon ground ginger

1 teaspoon ground cinnamon

1 pinch saffron strands

1 bay leaf

2 tablespoons low-sodium tomato purée

2 potatoes, peeled and diced

2 quarts water

6 plum tomatoes, diced

½ bunch cilantro leaves, chopped

Soak lentils overnight, rinse, and drain.

In a large nonstick saucepan, sauté the onions and garlic until light brown. Add the celery and cook until soft, about 3 minutes. Add the salt, pepper, turmeric, cumin, ginger, cinnamon, saffron, and bay leaf. Cook over low heat for ½ hour. Add the tomato purée, potatoes, lentils, and water. Cook over medium heat for 45 minutes, stirring occasionally. Add the plum tomatoes and cook over medium heat for 5 minutes. Remove bay leaf and garnish soup with the cilantro.

Nutrition Information (per 1-cup serving): 126 calories, less than 1g fat, less than 1g saturated fat, 0mg cholesterol, 9g protein, 6g fiber, 95mg sodium.

Sweet Potato and Kale Soup

MAKES 16 CUPS

2 pounds sweet potatoes, peeled and diced

1 onion, peeled and diced

1 carrot, peeled and diced

1 tablespoon fresh sage, finely chopped

2 tablespoons garlic, minced

2 quarts low-sodium vegetable stock (such as Pritikin recipe)

1 tablespoon low-sodium soy sauce

1 cup celery root, peeled and diced thin

4 bunches kale, washed and trimmed

In a stockpot, add all ingredients except the kale. Cook over medium heat, stirring occasionally, until all ingredients are soft, about 1 hour. Purée soup in a food processor and return to pot. Add the kale, and cook over medium heat for 15 minutes more.

Nutrition Information (per 1-cup serving): 68 calories, less than 1g fat, 0g saturated fat, 0mg cholesterol, 2g protein, 3g fiber, 85mg sodium.

Tomato Saffron Soup with Orange Essence

MAKES 8 CUPS

¼ cup chopped garlic

1 onion, puréed in food processor

½ small fennel bulb, diced*

About 15 saffron threads

½ cup white wine

½ cup orange juice

¼ bunch thyme, leaves picked and chopped

14 ounces low-sodium tomato purée

14 ounces whole peeled tomatoes, crushed by hand

½ gallon low-sodium vegetable stock (such as Pritikin recipe)

In a large stockpot, over medium heat, bring the garlic, onion, fennel, saffron, and wine to a low boil. Turn heat to a high simmer and cook mixture, stirring occasionally, until reduced by half. Add the orange juice, adjust heat and bring to a low boil, and reduce the mixture by half again on high-simmer heat. Add remaining ingredients. Bring to a boil and simmer for 1 hour. Serve hot.

Nutrition Information (per 1-cup serving): 55 calories, less than 1g fat, 0g saturated fat, 0mg cholesterol, 2g protein, 3g fiber, 36mg sodium.

---

* To prepare fennel, cut the stalks off the bulb to create a neat "package." Trim base of bulb and remove core and any discolored or tough outer leaves.

Pritikin Vegetable Stock

Pre-packaged vegetable stocks, even so-called low-sodium varieties, are often high in sodium—about 500 milligrams per cup. To dramatically cut your sodium intake (to 32 milligrams), make your own stock. It's pretty simple, as the guidelines below illustrate. This recipe freezes well, so one batch will last you a long time.

Basic guidelines for your stock:

- Always use celery, carrots, and onions.
- Other vegetables you can use include asparagus, squash, tomatoes, lettuce, mushrooms, zucchini, sweet peppers, green beans, potatoes, and peas. Never use old or yellowing vegetables.
- Be aware that vegetables from the cabbage family, including broccoli, cauliflower, and Brussels sprouts, will strongly flavor your stock. It is best not to use them, or to use only in small amounts.
- You can give your stock additional flavor by adding several whole cloves of garlic or the whole bulb, as well as 6 to 10 whole black peppercorns, 3 to 6 whole allspice, a few bay leaves, and fresh herbs, such as Italian parsley or thyme.

Assembling the stock:

- It is not necessary to peel the vegetables, even the garlic and onions. Rinse them well, cut some of the larger veggies into rough chunks, and fill your stockpot at least two-thirds to the top with assorted vegetables.
- Cover the vegetables completely with filtered water at least 2 inches above the vegetables. Bring the pot to a full boil and then immediately turn it down to a simmer. You will see occasional slow bubbles rising to the surface. Simmer your stock for approximately 2 to 2½ hours. Avoid stirring or it will turn cloudy.
- Turn off the heat and let the stock "rest" for about 30 minutes.

Strain your stock into a clean container and discard the vegetables.

- Freeze your stock in several convenient one-serving containers. Stock that's refrigerated should be used within four days.

Nutrition Information (per 1-cup serving): 30 calories, less than 1g fat, 0g saturated fat, 0mg cholesterol, 1g protein, 2g fiber, 31mg sodium.

Entrées

Aloo Phujia

Potatoes, onions, and tomatoes are given a spicy Indian kick. Serve as a side dish or over brown rice as a main dish.

SERVES 4

½ pound Idaho potatoes, peeled and diced

½ cup large-diced Vidalia onions

½ pound ripe tomatoes, diced (canned are okay)

¼ teaspoon cayenne pepper

¼ teaspoon turmeric

Pinch of cumin

1 tablespoon water

In a small covered stockpot, bring all ingredients to a boil over medium-high heat. Lower temperature to a simmer. Stirring occasionally, cook for 45 minutes, or until the potatoes are cooked and liquid is mostly evaporated. (If more water is needed to cook potatoes fully, add by small amounts. The liquid from the onions and tomatoes should do most of the cooking.)

Nutrition Information (per 1-cup serving): 63 calories, less than 1g fat, 0g saturated fat, 0mg cholesterol, 2g protein, 2g fiber, 7mg sodium.

Black Bean Chicken

SERVES 4

Four 4-ounce boneless, skinless chicken breasts

1 cup cooked black beans

½ cup diced red onion

½ cup corn, roasted*

Juice of 3 limes

1 tablespoon minced or sliced garlic

1 teaspoon cumin

1 teaspoon coriander

1 jalapeño pepper, finely chopped (seeds removed if you want to turn down the heat)

2 tablespoons chopped cilantro leaves

In a deep nonstick sauté pan, sear the chicken breasts on one side over medium-high heat until brown. Flip chicken over and add remaining ingredients, except the cilantro. Cover and cook for about 5 minutes at low heat. Check for doneness (chicken's internal temperature should be 165°F). Add the cilantro. Cook for 1 minute more. Serve hot.

Nutrition Information (per serving): 220 calories, 2g fat, less than 1g saturated fat, 66mg cholesterol, 31g protein, 5g fiber, 77mg sodium.

---

* To roast corn, pour kernels (thawed if from the freezer) on a nonstick cookie pan. Bake at 425°F for 20 minutes or until browned, stirring occasionally.

Braised Fish with Marsala, Shiitake Mushrooms, and Spinach

This recipe works well with halibut, monkfish, cobia, or sea bass.

SERVES 4

16 ounces fish, cut into 4-ounce portions

⅓ pound shiitake mushrooms, sliced

¼ cup sliced garlic

¼ cup sliced shallots

¼ cup Marsala wine

1 cup no-salt-added tomato sauce

1 teaspoon low-sodium soy sauce

½ teaspoon black peppercorns, ground

½ bunch basil, leaves chopped

½ bunch Italian parsley, leaves chopped

½ pound spinach leaves, cut into long, thin strips

Preheat oven to 400°F.

In a large nonstick skillet over high heat, sear the fish and mushrooms. When light brown, remove fish and add the garlic and shallots. When the garlic turns golden brown, loosen the brown bits of food on bottom of pan with the Marsala and reduce mixture by one-half, keeping temperature hot. Return fish to pan and add the tomato sauce, soy sauce, and black pepper. Place skillet in oven and bake until fish is cooked (about 3 minutes, depending on fish). Remove from oven and place on top of stove. Add the basil, parsley, and spinach. Cook until the spinach wilts. Serve immediately.

Nutrition Information (per serving): 177 calories, 1g fat, less than 1g saturated fat, 83mg cholesterol, 24g protein, 3g fiber, 186mg sodium.

Chicken with Cherry Tomatoes

This entrée pairs nicely with steamed new potatoes, mashed potatoes, or wild rice.

SERVES 4

Four 4-ounce boneless, skinless chicken breasts

1 teaspoon granulated garlic

1 teaspoon granulated onion

1 teaspoon salt-free lemon pepper

½ teaspoon chili powder

2 cups grape or cherry tomatoes, cut into halves

¼ cup low-sodium vegetable stock (such as Pritikin recipe)

Juice of 1 lemon

3 tablespoons chopped Italian parsley

Season the chicken with the garlic, onion, lemon pepper, and chili powder. In a nonstick skillet, sear both sides of the chicken breasts. Add the tomatoes, stock, and lemon juice. Simmer until chicken is fully cooked, about 5 minutes. Sprinkle each serving with parsley and serve immediately.

Nutrition Information (per serving): 148 calories, 2g fat, less than 1g saturated fat, 66mg cholesterol, 27g protein, 1g fiber, 82mg sodium.

Elk Chops with Garlic and Sage Crust

Grass-fed, free-range wild game such as buffalo (bison), elk, and moose are low in saturated fat, as low as skinless white poultry.

SERVES 4

   Four 5-ounce elk chops with the bone

   1 tablespoon minced garlic

   2 tablespoons chopped fresh sage leaves

   1 tablespoon chopped fresh rosemary leaves

   1 tablespoon juniper berries, ground

   1 teaspoon ground black pepper

   1 tablespoon ground coriander

Turn on broiler. Mix all the spices together. Coat the elk chops with spices. Place under a hot broiler for 2 minutes. Flip and cook for 1½ minutes more.

Nutrition Information (per serving): 168 calories, 2g fat, less than 1g saturated fat, 78mg cholesterol, 35g protein, 1g fiber, 83mg sodium.

Enchilada Bake

SERVES 4

¼ cup pico de gallo, puréed

½ cup canned red beans, no-salt-added (or rinsed to remove salt)

½ jalapeño pepper (optional), seeds removed

¼ cup chopped vegetarian meat substitute, such as So Soya (www.sosoya.com)

1 teaspoon cumin seeds, toasted and ground (see page 185)

Eight 6-inch corn tortillas, no added salt

1½ cups red chile sauce

Preheat oven to 350°F.

In a food processor, blend the pico de gallo, beans, jalapeño, meat substitute, and cumin until coarse.

Lay out the tortillas. Place one spoonful of bean mixture on the left side of each tortilla. Roll tortillas up. Place tortillas in a baking dish and pour red chile sauce over the top. Cover and bake for 10 minutes. Uncover and bake for 3 minutes more.

Nutrition Information (per 2-tortilla serving): 190 calories, 2g fat, less than 1g saturated fat, 0mg cholesterol, 10g protein, 7g fiber, 47mg sodium.

Fish en Papillote

Our Pritikin chefs often use whitefish or salmon in this recipe; shrimp and scallops are good choices, too.

SERVES 4

Parchment paper

Four 4-ounce servings of seafood

2 tomatoes, chopped

1 tablespoon fresh thyme leaves

1 red onion, chopped

2 tablespoons chopped fresh dill

¼ teaspoon black peppercorns, ground

½ cup white wine

Preheat oven to 400°F.

Cut four large rectangles of parchment paper and fold in half; unfold. Set aside.

Marinate the fish in remaining ingredients. Place fish in parchment paper, and top with the vegetables and herbs from the marinade. Fold top half of parchment paper over fish and crimp to seal. Place on two baking sheets. Bake until done, about 10 minutes. Open the top of each paper and serve immediately.

Nutrition Information (per serving): 157 calories, 1g fat, less than 1g saturated fat, 83mg cholesterol, 22g protein, 2g fiber, 105mg sodium.

Garden-Fresh Pan-Roasted Chicken Breast

SERVES 4

Four 4-ounce boneless, skinless chicken breasts

½ cup orange juice

1 tablespoon chopped fresh rosemary

1 pint grape tomatoes

1 large red onion, diced

1 large zucchini, diced

1 teaspoon chopped garlic

1 bunch asparagus, ends trimmed

1 teaspoon black pepper

1 tablespoon fresh basil leaves, chopped

Place the chicken breasts in a large nonstick skillet. Cook on one side for 2 minutes over medium-high heat. Add remaining ingredients, except the asparagus, pepper, and basil. Cover and lower heat to medium-low. Cook for 2 minutes. Flip chicken breasts. Add the asparagus and pepper, and cook for 2 more minutes. Add the basil. Serve immediately.

Nutrition Information (per serving): 200 calories, 2g fat, less than 1g saturated fat, 66mg cholesterol, 30g protein, 4g fiber, 87mg sodium.

Italian White Bean and Spinach Stew

MAKES ABOUT 4 CUPS

  1 cup finely diced red onion
  ¼ cup chopped garlic
  1 cup sliced red bell pepper
  ½ cup white wine
  8 fresh Roma tomatoes, seeded, finely chopped
  2 cups cooked white beans (if using canned beans, choose "no salt added" varieties
       or rinse and drain to remove sodium)
  2 tablespoons balsamic vinegar
  1 tablespoon low-sodium soy sauce
  ¾ teaspoon black pepper
  ½ cup fresh basil, leaves chopped
  1 pound fresh spinach, leaves picked, washed, and sliced

In a large stockpot, cook the onions, garlic, and red bell pepper in the white wine at medium-high heat for about 10 minutes. Add the tomatoes and white beans. Mix well and cook for another 20 minutes at medium to medium-low heat, stirring occasionally. Add the vinegar, soy sauce, black pepper, basil, and spinach. Cook until the spinach wilts. Serve immediately.

Nutrition Information (per 1-cup serving): 243 calories, 1g fat, less than 1g saturated fat, 0mg cholesterol, 15g protein, 11g fiber, 241mg sodium.

Meatless Meatballs

These meatballs are the most popular vegetarian dish among our guests at the Pritikin Longevity Center. You can freeze them, so double or triple the batch and save for nights when you'd rather not cook. Blend the meatballs with Fresh Tomato Sauce (see recipe on page 191) and ladle over whole-wheat pasta.

SERVES 4

    1 pound meat substitute*
    1 cup whole-wheat bread crumbs
    ½ teaspoon black peppercorns, ground
    2 teaspoons dried oregano
    2 tablespoons fresh basil leaves, cut in thin strips or shredded
    ½ onion, minced
    ½ cup Egg Beaters

Preheat oven to 350°F.

Mix all ingredients together. Mold into 12 balls. On a nonstick baking sheet, bake for 25 minutes.

Nutrition Information (per 3-meatball serving): 306 calories, 5g fat, 0g saturated fat, 0mg cholesterol, 34g protein, 13g fiber, 236mg sodium.

---

* Our chefs use a meat substitute from www.abfoodsllc.com. To order, call 800-822-3100 and ask for the special "beef" blend for the Pritikin Program. Another good meat substitute is So Soya (www.sosoya.com).

Pan-Roasted Lemon Ginger Salmon

SERVES 4

1 pound salmon, sliced into 4 portions

1 tablespoon chopped garlic

1 teaspoon paprika

1 tablespoon chopped fresh ginger

4 stalks lemongrass (Use only the bulb's soft interior; see note on page 200)

1 tablespoon lemon juice

To create marinade, purée all ingredients except the fish in a food processor.

Pour over fish and marinate for 20 minutes.

In a hot nonstick skillet, sear the salmon for 3 minutes on one side. Flip, cover, and cook on moderate to moderate-low heat until done, about 5 to 8 minutes depending on thickness of fish. Serve hot or cold.

Nutrition Information (per serving): 173 calories, 7g fat, 1g saturated fat, 62mg cholesterol, 23g protein, less than 1g fiber, 51mg sodium.

Penne with Charred Tomatoes and Oyster Mushrooms

SERVES 4

12 large tomatoes

3 cups sliced oyster mushrooms

1 cup finely sliced Vidalia onions

1 teaspoon finely chopped fresh rosemary

2 tablespoons minced garlic

¼ cup Splenda

½ teaspoon black peppercorns, freshly ground

2 tablespoons fresh basil leaves, sliced into very thin strips

1 teaspoon low-sodium soy sauce

4 cups whole-wheat penne, cooked with no salt

Preheat oven to 450°F. Place a nonstick baking sheet in oven and let heat for 10 minutes.

Meanwhile, cut the tomatoes in half. After removing baking sheet from oven, place tomatoes on sheet, cut sides facing up. Cook for 25 minutes, or until well browned. Remove from oven, let cool, and chop the tomatoes.

In a very hot nonstick skillet, brown the mushrooms for about 3 minutes. Add the onions, rosemary, and garlic. Cook for 1 minute more. Add remaining ingredients, including the cooked pasta. Cook for 2 minutes, or until all ingredients are heated through.

Nutrition Information (per 1-cup serving): 260 calories, 2g fat, less than 1g saturated fat, 0mg cholesterol, 14g protein, 14g fiber, 106mg sodium.

Seafood Romanesco Style

This recipe works well with cod, halibut, or salmon.

SERVES 4

1 pound fish, cut into 4-ounce portions

1 large red bell pepper, diced

½ large yellow bell pepper, diced

1 large onion, diced

8 cloves garlic, cut in large pieces

⅓ cup low-sodium vegetable stock (such as Pritikin recipe)

½ teaspoon low-sodium soy sauce

¼ teaspoon ground black peppercorns

⅓ cup white wine

½ bunch Italian parsley, leaves picked, washed, and chopped

In a large nonstick skillet, sauté the fish over medium heat. When browned, add the peppers, onions, and garlic. When the onions are translucent, add the stock, soy sauce, black pepper, and wine. Continue cooking. After the liquid has been reduced by half, turn heat to low and cook fish in sauce another 3 minutes. Garnish with the parsley. Serve hot.

Nutrition Information (per serving): 146 calories, 1g fat, less than 1g saturated fat, 83mg cholesterol, 22g protein, 2g fiber, 115mg sodium.

Seared Salmon with Arugula, Mushrooms, and Balsamic Vinegar

SERVES 4

½ teaspoon celery seed

2 juniper berries

¼ teaspoon dry basil

¼ teaspoon granulated onion

¼ teaspoon granulated garlic

¼ teaspoon chili powder

¼ teaspoon coriander

¼ teaspoon black peppercorns

1 tablespoon paprika

½ teaspoon chopped fresh thyme leaves

1 pound salmon, cut into four 4-ounce portions

1 pound assorted sliced mushrooms

10 ounces fresh arugula leaves, washed, dried, and sliced

4 tablespoons balsamic vinegar

Toast first nine ingredients together by placing them over high heat on the stove in a small heavy nonstick skillet. Toss them frequently until fragrant, about 2 to 4 minutes. Let cool. Add thyme. Grind all spices together. Coat the salmon in the spices.

In a hot skillet, cook the salmon and mushrooms on high heat for about 3 minutes. Flip salmon, cover, turn heat to low, and cook until done, about 5 minutes depending on thickness. Add the arugula and balsamic vinegar. Cover and cook on low heat for 2 minutes more. Serve immediately.

Nutrition Information (per serving): 221 calories, 8g fat, 1g saturated fat, 62mg cholesterol, 28g protein, 3g fiber, 80mg sodium.

Seared Whitefish with Rum and Thyme

SERVES 4

1 onion, peeled and diced

1 teaspoon cumin

1 teaspoon coriander

½ teaspoon black peppercorns, ground

2 teaspoons chopped fresh thyme leaves

1 cup orange juice

¼ cup lime juice

¼ cup dark rum

1 tablespoon cornstarch

2 tablespoons water

Four 4-ounce whitefish fillets

1 tablespoon chopped fresh cilantro leaves

Preheat oven to 450°F.

In a small stockpot, cook the onions over low heat until translucent, about 3 minutes. Add half portions of each of the spices and all of the orange juice, lime juice, and rum. Simmer sauce for 10 minutes. Thicken with cornstarch and water. Season the fish with the other half of the spices. In a very hot skillet, sear fish on one side for about 3 minutes. Put fish in oven in a baking dish to finish cooking, about 6 minutes. Add the cilantro to the sauce. Spoon sauce over fish.

Nutrition Information (per serving): 253 calories, 7g fat, 1g saturated fat, 68mg cholesterol, 23g protein, 2g fiber, 62mg sodium.

Spinach and Mushroom Crustless Quiche

SERVES 4

½ cup diced onion

2 tablespoons chopped garlic

24 ounces frozen chopped spinach, thawed and drained

8 ounces sliced fresh mushrooms

1 tablespoon granulated onion

1 tablespoon granulated garlic

¼ teaspoon ground black pepper

¼ cup egg whites

Pam or other oil spray

Preheat oven to 400°F.

In a large nonstick skillet, sauté the onion and garlic until brown. Add the spinach, mushrooms, granulated onion, granulated garlic, and black pepper, and cook until spinach is hot, about 2 to 4 minutes. Let quiche mixture cool in refrigerator.

When mixture is cool, mix in the egg whites. Spread mixture on a half-sheet pan lightly sprayed with Pam or other oil spray. Bake for 15 minutes. Let stand at room temperature for 10 minutes before cutting into serving sizes.

Nutrition Information (per serving): 100 calories, 2g fat, less than 1g saturated fat, 0mg cholesterol, 11g protein, 7g fiber, 155mg sodium.

Spinach-Stuffed Salmon with Mango Sauce

SERVES 4

Mango Sauce

1 mango, peeled and diced

½ cup plain nonfat yogurt

Juice of one lime

1 cup sliced oyster mushrooms

1 tablespoon sliced shallots

1 tablespoon chopped garlic

1 pound fresh spinach, chopped

Four 4-ounce salmon fillets, butterflied (cut crosswise and spread open flat)

4 thin slices pineapple

1 teaspoon paprika

½ teaspoon black peppercorns, ground

For the mango sauce: In a food processor, purée all ingredients until smooth. Chill.

In a hot nonstick skillet, sauté the mushrooms, shallots, and garlic until garlic is light brown. Add the spinach. Cook for 1 minute, and remove from heat.

In the butterflied salmon, layer the pineapple slices and the spinach mixture. Close salmon, and dust with the paprika and pepper. Lay skin side up in a hot skillet and cook over medium heat until bottom is cooked, about 3 minutes. Cover and lower heat. Cook for 8 more minutes. Serve with mango sauce.

Nutrition Information (per serving): 309 calories, 13g fat, 4g saturated fat, 57mg cholesterol, 30g protein, 5g fiber, 179mg sodium.

Tofu Italian

SERVES 4

1 large red bell pepper, diced

1 large yellow bell pepper, diced

1 large onion, diced

8 cloves garlic, cut in large pieces

½ cup low-sodium vegetable stock (such as Pritikin recipe)

½ teaspoon low-sodium soy sauce

¼ teaspoon black peppercorns, ground

½ cup white wine

1 pound firm tofu

½ bunch Italian parsley leaves, chopped

In a large nonstick skillet over medium heat, sauté the bell peppers, on-ions, and garlic. When the onions are translucent, add the stock, soy sauce, black pepper, and wine. Cook until liquid is reduced by half. Set sauce aside.

In a large nonstick skillet, sear the tofu on one side. Add the sauce to the skillet, and let the tofu cook in the sauce for 3 minutes. Garnish with the parsley. Serve hot.

Nutrition Information (per serving): 151 calories, 4g fat, 1g saturated fat, 0mg choles-terol, 10g protein, 3g fiber, 43mg sodium.

Snacks, Salads, and Side Dishes

In Chapter 8, we gave you our quick-and-easy snack recipes; here you'll find some additional ones for when you have a little more time to prepare them in advance.

Cabbage Salad with Coriander and Lemon

SERVES 4

½ head cabbage, sliced very thin

½ red onion, cut into long, thin strips

¼ cup chopped cilantro leaves

¼ cup finely chopped garlic

1 tablespoon coriander seeds

½ cup lemon juice

¼ cup white vinegar

½ teaspoon nutmeg

1 tablespoon Splenda

¼ teaspoon black peppercorns, ground

In a large bowl, mix all ingredients. Let sit for 1 hour before serving.

Nutrition Information (per 1-cup serving): 48 calories, less than 1g fat, less than 1g saturated fat, 0mg cholesterol, 2g protein, 3g fiber, 22mg sodium.

Carrot and Pineapple Salad

SERVES 4

2 carrots, shredded

½ pineapple, diced

Juice of 2 limes

1 tablespoon basil, cut into fine, thin strips

¼ teaspoon black peppercorns, ground

1 tablespoon mint, cut into fine, thin strips

1 tablespoon chopped chives

In a large bowl, mix all ingredients well and let sit for 10 minutes. Chill and serve cold.

Nutrition Information (per 1-cup serving): 43 calories, less than 1g fat, less than 1g saturated fat, 0mg cholesterol, less than 1g protein, 2g fiber, 17mg sodium.

Crispy Potato Skins

SERVES 4 (2 POTATO SKINS PER SERVING)

4 baked potatoes
¼ teaspoon garlic powder
¼ teaspoon onion powder
¼ teaspoon paprika

Preheat oven to 400°F.

Mix garlic, onion, and paprika together and set aside. Cut the potatoes in half lengthwise. Scoop out potatoes almost down to the skin. Place potato skins on a nonstick baking sheet. Sprinkle garlic mixture lightly over the skins. Bake for 10 minutes, or until crisp. (Use scooped-out center of potato for mashed potatoes or thickening soups.)

Nutrition Information (per serving): 88 calories, less than 1g fat, 0g saturated fat, 0mg cholesterol, 2g protein, 4g fiber, 9mg sodium.

Hummus Dip

This is great as a snack or appetizer. Serve it with raw vegetables or stuff into whole-wheat pita bread with fresh veggies.

SERVES 4

One 15-ounce can of garbanzo beans, no-salt-added, or rinsed and drained

¼ cup lemon juice (adjust according to taste)

1 tablespoon minced fresh garlic

2 tablespoons chopped Italian parsley

¼ cup chopped fresh dill

1 dash Tabasco sauce

⅛ teaspoon white pepper

½ cup chopped celery

In a food processor, purée all ingredients. If mixture is too thick, add 1 tablespoon of water.

Nutrition Information (per ½-cup serving): 185 calories, 3g fat, less than 1g saturated fat, 0mg cholesterol, 10g protein, 9g fiber, 23mg sodium.

Jicama and Red Pepper Slaw

SERVES 4

1 jicama, peeled

1 red bell pepper

¼ head red cabbage

6 chives

1 tablespoon Splenda

¼ cup brown rice vinegar

¼ teaspoon black peppercorns, ground

1 tablespoon lime juice

1 tablespoon orange juice

Slice the jicama, red bell pepper, and cabbage into long thin strips. Cut the chives into thirds. In a large bowl, mix remaining ingredients. Mix all ingredients together. Let sit for 10 minutes before serving.

Nutrition Information (per 1-cup serving): 77 calories, less than 1g fat, 0g saturated fat, 0mg cholesterol, 2g protein, 7g fiber, 19mg sodium.

Leek, Cauliflower, Green Bean, and Celery Salad

SERVES 4

½ head cauliflower, blanched and cut into bite-size pieces

1 cup green beans, blanched and diced

¼ cup diced celery

¼ cup chopped leeks

¼ cup diced red bell pepper

1 tablespoon minced Italian parsley

¼ cup white balsamic vinegar

1 teaspoon celery seeds

1 teaspoon paprika

1 tablespoon frozen apple juice concentrate

1 teaspoon low-sodium Dijon mustard

¼ cup fat-free sour cream

In a large bowl, mix all ingredients together. Chill and serve cold.

Nutrition Information (per 1-cup serving): 46 calories, less than 1g fat, 0g saturated fat, 0mg cholesterol, 2g protein, 3g fiber, 38mg sodium.

Malbulha

Middle Eastern in origin, malbulha is a tomato-pepper salad, dip, or spread.

SERVES 4

1 tablespoon minced garlic

½ onion, peeled and diced

2 red bell peppers, seeds removed and diced

½ cup canned diced tomatoes, low-sodium or no-salt-added

¼ cup tomato purée

¼ cup lemon juice

1 teaspoon cumin seeds, toasted and ground*

1 teaspoon coriander seeds, toasted and ground*

¼ teaspoon black peppercorns, ground

¼ teaspoon paprika

¼ teaspoon cayenne pepper or ½ jalapeño pepper, diced

In a hot stockpot, sauté the garlic and onions until light brown. Add remaining ingredients and lower heat. Cook for 30 minutes, stirring regularly. Cool before serving.

Nutrition Information (per ½-cup serving): 40 calories, less than 1g fat, 0g saturated fat, 0mg cholesterol, 2g protein, 2g fiber, 13mg sodium.

---

* To toast seeds, place them over high heat on the stove in a small heavy skillet. Toss them frequently until fragrant, about 2 to 4 minutes.

Potato Corn Cakes

SERVES 4

½ cup Egg Beaters

½ cup quick-cooking polenta

¼ cup cornstarch

3 ears of corn, kernels removed (Frozen corn kernels, thawed, will work, but not as well. Use 1½ cups.)

2 baked potatoes, peeled and shredded

½ onion, peeled and diced

¼ cup sliced scallions

1 teaspoon chopped garlic

1 teaspoon chopped fresh thyme leaves

1 teaspoon chopped fresh sage leaves

Pam or other oil spray

Preheat oven to 400°F.

Whisk together the Egg Beaters, polenta, and cornstarch until well mixed, about 3 minutes. In a large bowl, mix all remaining ingredients. Fold Egg Beaters mixture into potato mixture. Form into 4 patties.

In a hot skillet, lightly spray Pam or other oil spray. Add the patties and cook until brown. Flip and brown other side. Put patties on baking dish and bake for 10 minutes. Serve hot.

Nutrition Information (per corn patty): 271 calories, 1g fat, less than 1g saturated fat, 0mg cholesterol, 10g protein, 7g fiber, 84mg sodium.

Sage-Rubbed Potatoes

SERVES 4

2 large potatoes, washed and sliced into wedges

Pam or other oil spray

¼ cup garlic cloves

2 tablespoons fresh sage leaves

1 tablespoon fresh rosemary leaves

Juice and zest of 2 lemons

1 tablespoon fresh Italian parsley leaves

Juice of 1 lime

Preheat oven to 450°F.

Steam the potato wedges until half cooked, about 10 minutes. Let cool.

Spray a sheet pan lightly with Pam or other oil spray. Place the potatoes on the pan and bake for 15 to 20 minutes, or until cooked through and crispy.

While potatoes are baking, purée the garlic, sage, rosemary, lemon juice, lemon zest, and parsley in a food processor. In a large bowl, mix the garlic paste with the lime juice.

After potatoes have finished baking, toss them in the garlic/lime mixture and serve.

Nutrition Information (per serving): 39 calories, less than 1g fat, 0g saturated fat, 0mg cholesterol, 2g protein, 3g fiber, 8mg sodium.

Spicy Cucumbers

SERVES 4

    2 large cucumbers, peeled, seeds removed, and sliced

    ½ tablespoon paprika

    Pinch cayenne pepper

    Pinch black peppercorns, ground

    ½ cup fresh lemon juice

In a large bowl, mix all ingredients together. Let sit for 5 minutes and serve.

Nutrition Information (per serving): 16 calories, less than 1g fat, 0g saturated fat, 0mg cholesterol, less than 1g protein, less than 1g fiber, 2mg sodium.

Sweet Potato and Apple Salad

This recipe is always a hit in cooking class at the Pritikin Longevity Center. It's a great dessert as well as salad. For dessert, give it a nice chill by slipping it into the freezer just before you sit down for your main course. By dessert time, it will be ready to serve.

SERVES 4

3 cups cooked diced sweet potatoes

1 cup diced apple

1 tablespoon lemon juice

2 ounces fat-free sour cream

½ teaspoon cinnamon

½ tablespoon frozen apple juice concentrate

½ teaspoon vanilla extract

In a large bowl, mix all ingredients well. Refrigerate for 30 minutes before serving.

Nutrition Information (per 1 cup serving): 119 calories, less than 1g fat, less than 1g saturated fat, 1mg cholesterol, 2g protein, 4g fiber, 53mg sodium.

Tabouli

Tabouli is a Middle Eastern dish, often eaten by scooping it up in lettuce leaves. The chefs at the Pritikin Longevity Center serve it as a salad or side dish.

SERVES 4

¾ cup bulgur wheat

1 to 1½ cups hot water

Juice of 2 lemons

2 teaspoons rice vinegar

1 teaspoon minced garlic

½ cup minced tomatoes

¼ cup minced green onions

½ cup minced Italian parsley

½ cup minced mint

1 teaspoon paprika

½ teaspoon black peppercorns, ground

Soak the bulgur in enough hot water to cover for 30 minutes.

In a large bowl, combine bulgur with remaining ingredients and chill well.

Nutrition Information (per 1-cup serving): 110 calories, less than 1g fat, 0g saturated fat, 0mg cholesterol, 4g protein, 6g fiber, 14mg sodium.

Thai Coleslaw

SERVES 4

Dressing

½ cup brown rice vinegar

1 tablespoon apple juice concentrate

1 tablespoon basil, cut in thin strips or shreds

¼ cup peeled and minced ginger

2 teaspoons minced garlic

1 teaspoon minced dill

1 teaspoon minced lemongrass (use only bulb's soft interior)

1 teaspoon low-sodium Dijon mustard

Vegetables

1½ cups shredded green cabbage

1½ cups shredded red cabbage

1 cup rinsed and shredded carrots

In a blender or food processor, blend all dressing ingredients.

In a large bowl, combine dressing with vegetables. Refrigerate for one hour before serving.

Nutrition Information (per serving): 52 calories, less than 1g fat, 0g saturated fat, 0mg cholesterol, 2g protein, 3g fiber, 70mg sodium.

Tomato and Rosemary Salad

SERVES 4

4 ripe tomatoes, diced

1 tablespoon rosemary, leaves picked and chopped

1 tablespoon minced garlic

¼ teaspoon black peppercorns, ground

¼ cup chopped Italian parsley leaves

Juice of 2 lemons

1 teaspoon oregano

In a hot skillet, sear the tomatoes with the rosemary and garlic. When tomatoes are just beginning to break down, stir in remaining ingredients. Serve immediately.

Nutrition Information (per 1-cup serving): 47 calories, less than 1g fat, 0g saturated fat, 0mg cholesterol, 2g protein, 3g fiber, 14mg sodium.

Desserts

Apple Turnovers

SERVES 4

3 large Granny Smith apples, peeled, cored, and sliced

½ teaspoon cinnamon

Juice of 1 lemon

¼ cup raisins

1 pinch cloves

1 teaspoon vanilla extract

1 teaspoon Splenda

1 tablespoon cornstarch

2 whole-wheat, low-sodium lavash breads, each cut in half

Sauce

½ cup low-fat vanilla-flavored soymilk

1 teaspoon vanilla extract

½ cup fat-free sour cream

Preheat oven to 350°F.

In a large bowl, toss all turnover ingredients, except the lavash breads, together and bake in a Pyrex dish for 30 minutes.

Meanwhile, mix all sauce ingredients well and chill.

Cool apple mixture, then spread on lavash breads. Roll up. Spoon a little sauce on each serving plate. Lay turnovers on top. Serve cold.

Nutrition Information (per turnover): 165 calories, 1g fat, less than 1g saturated fat, 3mg cholesterol, 5g protein, 4g fiber, 114mg sodium.

Cherries Jubilee

SERVES 4

½ cinnamon stick

2 ounces water

½ tablespoon brandy

1 tablespoon Splenda

½ tablespoon cornstarch mixed with 1 tablespoon water

1 pound whole pitted dark tart cherries (fresh or frozen)

In a hot stockpot, add the cinnamon, water, brandy, and Splenda. Bring to a boil, turn heat down, and simmer for 10 minutes. Thicken by adding the cornstarch. Add the cherries. Remove cinnamon stick. Simmer for 5 minutes more.

Nutrition Information (per ½-cup serving): 107 calories, 0g fat, 0g saturated fat, 0mg cholesterol, 2g protein, less than 1g fiber, less than 1mg sodium.

Crustless Cherry Pie

SERVES 4

2 cups frozen pitted cherries

1 tablespoon frozen apple juice concentrate

½ tablespoon lemon juice

1½ tablespoons cornstarch

½ tablespoon vanilla extract

¼ cup rolled oats

Preheat oven to 350°F.

In a large bowl, mix all ingredients except the oats. Place the cherry mixture in ramekins. (Or, if you use larger pans, increase baking time.) Sprinkle the oats on top. Bake for 25 minutes. Let cool before serving.

Nutrition Information (per 4-ounce serving): 130 calories, 2g fat, less than 1g saturated fat, 0mg cholesterol, 4g protein, 3g fiber, 2mg sodium.

Chocolate Mousse

SERVES 4

4 tablespoons Hershey's unsweetened cocoa powder

¼ cup hot water

12 ounces extra-firm silken tofu

¼ cup Splenda

2 teaspoons vanilla extract

4 raspberries (optional)

In a small stainless steel bowl, combine the cocoa powder and hot water. Pour enough water to cover stainless steel bowl halfway into a pot and bring to a light simmer. Place the bowl in water and cook slowly for 5 minutes, or until the cocoa mixture is the consistency of fudge.

In a food processor, blend the tofu for 1 minute. Add the cocoa fudge, Splenda, and vanilla extract. Blend until smooth.

Spoon into serving glasses, cool, and chill before serving. Garnish with a raspberry, if desired.

Nutrition Information (per serving): 104 calories, 4g fat, 2g saturated fat, 0mg cholesterol, 12g protein, 9g fiber, 90mg sodium.

Jewel of Fruit Pie

SERVES 4

1 cup rolled oats

1 banana, sliced crosswise

1 pint strawberries, washed, hulled, and sliced

1 Granny Smith apple, peeled, cored, and sliced medium thin

½ teaspoon vanilla extract

1 pinch cinnamon

1 tablespoon date sugar

1 pinch nutmeg

¼ cup water

Preheat oven to 350°F.

Grind ¾ cup of the oats in a food processor. Pack firmly on bottom of 9" x 9" Pyrex baking dish and bake for 2 minutes. Let cool. Grind the remaining ¼ cup of oats and mix with remaining ingredients. Pour mixture very gently over crust and bake for 30 minutes. Cool and serve.

Nutrition Information (per 4-ounce slice): 147 calories, 2g fat, less than 1g saturated fat, 0mg cholesterol, 3g protein, 4g fiber, 2mg sodium.

Mango Parfait

SERVES 4

2 mangoes, peeled, sliced, and puréed (should make about 1½ cups of purée)

2 cups nonfat plain yogurt

1 tablespoon Splenda

¼ tablespoon frozen apple juice concentrate

½ cup raspberries

4 mint sprigs and 4 mango slices

In a large mixing bowl, combine the mango purée and yogurt. Add the Splenda and apple juice concentrate. Whisk until smooth.

Place the raspberries on the bottoms of 4 white wineglasses or 4 stemmed water glasses. Fill until two-thirds full with the mango/yogurt mixture. Place glasses in freezer for approximately 2 hours, or until parfaits are half frozen. Garnish each glass with a mint sprig and a mango slice. Serve immediately.

Nutrition Information (per ½-cup serving): 142 calories, less than 1g fat, 0g saturated fat, 3mg cholesterol, 7g protein, 3g fiber, 97mg sodium.

Strawberry Yogurt Swirl

SERVES 4

1 cup whole strawberries, washed and stems removed

1 ripe banana

1 cup plain nonfat yogurt

½ teaspoon vanilla

½ tablespoon Splenda

1 cup blueberries

In a blender, blend the strawberries.

In a large bowl, mash the banana into the yogurt with a whisk. Combine all ingredients except the blueberries. Fold in the blueberries. Chill and serve cold.

Nutrition Information (per ¾-cup serving): 94 calories, less than 1g fat, 0g saturated fat, 1mg cholesterol, 4g protein, 3g fiber, 48mg sodium.

Tia Maria Parfait

SERVES 4

4 tablespoons Tia Maria coffee liqueur

½ teaspoon vanilla extract

2 cups fat-free, sugar-free vanilla ice cream

¼ cup fresh raspberries

4 sprigs mint leaves

In a small saucepan over moderate heat, reduce the Tia Maria and vanilla extract to half their amount and let cool.

In 4 parfait glasses, pour equal amounts of the Tia Maria reduction. In each glass, place one scoop of ice cream. Use a teaspoon to gently press down ice cream. (The Tia Maria will float to the top.) Garnish with the raspberries and mint leaves. Serve immediately.

Nutritional Information (per ½-cup serving): 220 calories, less than 1g fat, 0g saturated fat, 0mg cholesterol, 5g protein, 2g fiber, 111mg sodium.

PART FOUR

Two-Week
Sample Menu

Below is a sample two-week meal plan that shows how you can easily incorporate all the healthy eating methods you learned in this book. See Appendix C for a complete nutrition analysis of this two-week plan.

DAY 1

Breakfast

- Cook in the microwave:
  ½ cup oatmeal
  1 cup nonfat milk
- Top with ½ banana and ½ cup blueberries
- 1 cup tea or coffee with 1 tablespoon nonfat milk or soymilk and 1 packet of sugar substitute (a good choice is Splenda)

Midmorning Snack

- 1 apple
- 1 six-inch steamed corn tortilla with:
  ¼ cup vegetables (such as onions, green bell peppers, and mushrooms)
  2 tablespoons no-added-salt salsa
  Warm the tortilla between slightly moistened towels in the microwave for about 1 minute, then top with veggies and salsa, and fold.

Lunch

- 2 cups mixed greens with 1 cup of other veggies (such as carrots and tomatoes), dressed with balsamic vinegar and topped with 1 tablespoon chopped walnuts

- 1 cup hearty black bean soup (See recipes or use a no-salt-added, fat-free canned variety like Healthy Valley or frozen variety like Tabatchnick.)
- 1 ear of corn on the cob with pinch (less than ¼ teaspoon) salt

Midafternoon Snack

- 6 ounces nonfat plain or no-sugar-added yogurt (good choices include Dannon Light & Fit, Stonyfield Farm, and fat-free, plain Greek-style yogurts such as Oikos and Fage)
- 1 cup grapes

Dinner

- Tomato salad with:
  2 cups tomatoes
  1 tablespoon fresh basil
  ½ sliced cucumber
  2 tablespoons red wine vinegar
  ¼ avocado, sliced
- 4 ounces fresh grilled seafood (See recipes. When dining out, ask that your seafood not be basted or bathed in calorie-dense ingredients like oil and butter.)
- 1 baked potato with 2 tablespoons fat-free sour cream
- 1 cup steamed broccoli with 1 teaspoon garlic and 1 teaspoon lemon juice

Dessert

- 1 cup fresh strawberries in 1 tablespoon Marsala wine

DAY 2

Breakfast

- 3-egg-white omelet with:
  2 tablespoons low-fat ricotta cheese
  ¼ cup grilled zucchini
  ¼ cup grilled onion
  ½ cup grilled red bell peppers
- ½ grapefruit
- 1 cup hot cocoa with nonfat milk or soymilk, 1 tablespoon cocoa powder, and 1 packet sugar substitute

Midmorning Snack

- 1 cup diced watermelon

Lunch

- 1 cup gazpacho
- 2 cups baby spinach with ⅓ teaspoon wasabi (to taste) and 2 tablespoons rice vinegar
- Fresh roasted turkey breast sandwich (3 ounces) on low-sodium whole-grain bread (2 slices) with bean sprouts, tomato slices, 1 tablespoon stone-ground mustard, and 1 teaspoon nonfat mayonnaise
- 1 cup fresh fruit

Midafternoon Snack

- 2 cups air-popped popcorn (A good ready-made brand is Bearito's no-salt, no-oil variety.)
- 1 red bell pepper, sliced

Dinner

- 2 cups mixed greens with ½ cup cannellini beans, ¼ of an avocado, and 2 tablespoons vinegar and 1 teaspoon canola oil

- 1 cup bean soup
- Penne with Charred Tomatoes and Oyster Mushrooms (page 217) (When dining out, request pasta primavera without cheese or butter and minimal oil, preferably none.)
- 2 cups steamed carrots and broccoli (In restaurants, ask for a double or triple order of vegetables.)

Dessert

- Chocolate Mousse (page 241)

DAY 3

Breakfast

- 1 cup hot cereal, such as oatmeal, cracked wheat, whole grain, or barley, made with 1 cup nonfat milk and 1 cup sliced fresh fruit (There are many good brands of hot cereals. Just make sure you buy one with no added salt or sugar.)
- ½ cup 100% fruit juice diluted with ½ cup sparkling or still water
- 1 cup tea or coffee with 1 tablespoon nonfat milk or soymilk and 1 packet of sugar substitute (a good choice is Splenda)

Midmorning Snack

- 6 whole-wheat low-sodium crackers (Good brand choices for crackers are Kavli, Wasa, FINN Crisp, Rye-Crisp, and RyVita.)
- ½ cup Red Pepper Dip
  Mix ⅓ cup canned roasted peppers with 1 tablespoon fat-free sour cream, 1 tablespoon chopped fresh basil, and 1 tablespoon balsamic vinegar in blender.

Lunch

- 2 cups mixed greens with 2 tablespoons flavored vinegar (no sugar, no salt added; good choices include Consorzio Raspberry or Mango and Mr. Spice Honey Mustard) and 1 teaspoon canola oil.
- 1 veggie burger (such as Gardenburger Garden Vegan) with grilled onions, lettuce, tomato, and low-sodium mustard (such as Westbrae) on ½ whole-grain, low-sodium hamburger bun (such as Food For Life's Ezekiel) topped with ¼ avocado

Midafternoon Snack

- 1 cup celery sticks with ½ cup bean dip (Good choices for ready-made, low-sodium bean dip brands include Bearitos and Guiltless Gourmet.)

- ½ cup fresh, cut-up fruit from a supermarket salad bar with 1 cup plain yogurt, nonfat

Dinner

- 1 cup Chinese Tomato Soup
  Combine no-salt-added canned tomatoes, onion, garlic, bok choy, and bean sprouts, seasoned with curry, chili powder, and a teaspoon of low-sodium soy sauce. Bring to a boil on stovetop and simmer at moderate heat for about 20 minutes.
- Greek salad with:
  1 cup romaine lettice
  1 cup red leaf lettuce
  ¼ cup sliced cucumber
  1 sliced Roma tomato
  2 tablespoons fresh lemon juice
  ⅛ ounce nonfat or low-fat feta cheese
- Snapper (3.5 ounces) steamed in foil. Season fish with a no-salt-added blackened blend of seasonings, wrap fish in foil, place on baking sheet, and bake in pre-heated oven at 350°F for 10 to 15 minutes, checking for doneness (internal temperature should reach 145°F). Season with 1 teaspoon low-sodium soy sauce. Serve fish with 1 cup of cooked wild rice.

Dessert

- No-sugar-added frozen 100% fruit bar

DAY 4

Breakfast

- Shredded wheat or crisp brown rice cereal, such as Erewhon, with 1 cup nonfat milk and 1 cup fresh strawberries
- 1 cup tea or coffee with 1 tablespoon nonfat milk or soymilk and 1 packet of sugar substitute

Midmorning Snack

- Spicy Cucumbers

  Mix ½ cup cucumbers with fresh lemon juice, paprika, and cayenne pepper to taste
- 1 fresh orange
- 1 ounce walnuts

Lunch

- 2 cups tomato salad topped with freshly chopped basil leaves, 2 tablespoons balsamic vinegar and 1½ teaspoons canola oil
- 1 Vegetable Quesadilla with:

  1½ cups mixed vegetables

  One 6-inch whole-wheat tortilla

  Bake at 450°F in a pan sprayed with a little no-stick cooking spray until tortilla browns.
- 1 ear of corn on the cob with a pinch (less than ¼ teaspoon) salt

Midafternoon Snack

- 1 cup sliced jicama
- 10 baked tortilla chips with ½ cup mango and black bean salsa

  To make salsa, combine 2 tablespoons cubed fresh mango, 2 tablespoons low-sodium salsa, and ¼ cup black beans, no salt added, drained and rinsed. (A good brand choice for tortilla chips is baked, no-salt-added Guiltless Gourmet.)

Dinner

- 2 cups mixed greens dressed with 1 tablespoon fat-free plain yogurt blended with 1 tablespoon Dijon mustard
- Spiced Lentil Soup (page 201)
- 3.5 ounces roasted bison sirloin or tenderloin cut
- 8 ounces Sage-Rubbed Potatoes (page 232) and horseradish cream
  To make horseradish cream, combine 1 tablespoon horseradish with 1 tablespoon fat-free sour cream or fat-free plain yogurt.

Dessert

- ½ cup fat-free, sugar-free ice cream (Good brand choices are Breyers and Edy's.)

DAY 5

Breakfast

- ½ whole-wheat bagel with 2 tablespoons low-fat cream cheese and 2 teaspoons fresh herbs
- 1 cup fresh fruit
- 1 cup tea or coffee with 1 tablespoon nonfat milk or soymilk and 1 packet of sugar substitute

Midmorning Snack

- 2 cups fresh pre-washed, pre-cut vegetables with ½ cup pinto bean dip.

  To make bean dip, combine ⅓ cup no-salt-added pinto beans, 2 tablespoons chopped red onion, cilantro, and lime juice to taste; blend in a food processor.

Lunch

- 1 grilled vegetable pizza (without cheese)

  6-inch round crust made with store-bought ready-to-roll-out whole-wheat pizza dough with 1½ cups fresh vegetables
- Stir-fry with 4 ounces of firm tofu and 1 cup broccoli, spiced with Tabasco sauce

Midafternoon Snack

- Mix together:

  ⅓ cup garbanzo beans

  ⅓ cup cauliflower florets

  ⅓ cup green beans

  ¼ cup nonfat plain yogurt

  ¼ cup grapes

Dinner

- 2 cups mixed greens with ½ cup cooked whole-wheat couscous, 2 tablespoons red onion, 1 tablespoon low-sodium soy sauce and 1 teaspoon canola oil
- 4 ounces Braised Fish with Marsala, Shiitake Mushrooms, and Spinach (page 208)
- 1 cup baked sweet potato fries

Dessert

- 1 cup fresh mixed berries

DAY 6

Breakfast

- 2 whole-wheat buttermilk pancakes or waffles with 1 cup fresh berries
- 1 cup plain yogurt, nonfat
- ½ cup 100% fruit juice diluted with ½ cup sparkling or still water
- 1 cup tea or coffee with 1 tablespoon nonfat milk or soymilk and 1 packet of sugar substitute

Midmorning Snack

- 1 cup cherry tomatoes with ¼ cup Hummus Dip (page 227)

Lunch

- 1 cup Sweet Potato and Kale Soup (page 202), add 1 teaspoon low-sodium soy sauce to taste
- 4 ounces canned low-sodium salmon with 1 teaspoon fresh dill, ¼ cup sliced cucumber, and 1 tablespoon chopped onion on 1 whole-wheat, low-sodium pita pocket.
- 1 apple

Midafternoon Snack

- ½ cup grated carrots mixed with ½ cup pineapple slices
- 1 slice whole-wheat toast with 1 tablespoon almond butter (go easy on the almond butter if you're trying to lose weight; it is high in calories.)

Dinner

- 2 cups baby spinach with 2 tablespoons Creamy-Style House Dressing (page 182)
- 1 cup vegetable or bean soup
- Enchilada Bake (page 211)

Dessert

- Berry Mousse

  Blend ½ cup berries, ½ cup silken tofu, 1 teaspoon Splenda, and ½ teaspoon vanilla extract to taste; serve cold.

DAY 7

Breakfast

- Cook in the microwave:
  ½ cup oatmeal
  1 cup nonfat milk
- Top with ½ banana
- 1 cup tea or coffee with 1 tablespoon nonfat milk or soymilk and 1 packet of sugar substitute

Midmorning Snack

- 1 cup fresh fruit
- 1 cup nonfat vanilla yogurt, no-sugar-added (A good brand is Dannon Light & Fit.)

Lunch

- 1 cup Corn Chowder (page 196)
- Garden-Fresh Vegetable Stir Fry
  Add 1½ teaspoon dark sesame oil to a heated wok and toss in a bag of cut, washed Asian-style veggies (3 cups); season with chili garlic sauce and ¾ tablespoon low-sodium soy sauce to taste.

Midafternoon Snack

- 2 Crispy Potato Skins (page 226)

Dinner

- 2 cups mixed greens with ½ cup tomatoes and ½ cup cucumbers, dressed with 2 tablespoons balsamic vinegar
- Minestrone
  Add leftover vegetables to a can of no-salt-added tomato sauce, a can of no-salt-added red beans, cooked whole-wheat pasta, and salt-free Italian seasoning. Heat and serve.

- 3.5 ounces slow-roasted Cornish hen (serve with skin removed) roasted with navy beans, tomatoes, and red wine, garnished with chopped fresh Italian parsley and basil
- 1 cup cooked quinoa

Dessert

- 1 cup Strawberry Yogurt Swirl (page 244)

DAY 8

Breakfast

- 3-egg-white-omelet with:
  2 tablespoons low-fat ricotta cheese
  ¼ cup grilled zucchini
  ¼ cup grilled onion
  ½ cup grilled red bell peppers
- ½ whole-grain English muffin with 1 teaspoon 100% fruit spread
- 1 cup tea or coffee with 1 tablespoon nonfat milk or soymilk and 1 packet of sugar substitute

Midmorning Snack

- 1 cup pre-cut, pre-sliced fruit, such as honeydew or pineapple
- 1 ounce 100% whole-wheat pretzels (Good brand choices are Barbara's and Martin's; check nutrition label for 1-ounce serving size. Pretzels are calorie-dense.)
- ½ cup plain yogurt, nonfat

Lunch

- 1 cup Eight Bean Soup (page 197)
- Italian Veggie Roll-Up
  Roast or grill 1½ cups of vegetables (such as eggplant, zucchini, squash, and red bell pepper slices) and roll in 1 whole-wheat wrap. (Good choices are Garden of Eatin' and Thin Thin.)

Midafternoon Snack

- 1 cup of cherry tomatoes with ¼ cup vegetable dip
  To make dip, blend steamed vegetables with fat-free sour cream and herbs in a food processor.

Dinner

- 2 cups of mixed greens with 2 tablespoons berry vinaigrette (A good choice is Consorzio Raspberry, or make your own by purée-ing white vinegar, strawberries, dill, garlic, apple juice, and a little vanilla extract.)
- 1 cup vegetable soup

  Combine any leftover vegetables you have with Knudsen Very Veggie Juice, Low Sodium, and your favorite salt-free blend of spices, and heat.
- Shrimp Fajitas:

  3.5 ounces cooked shrimp, cooked in 1 teaspoon canola oil

  ¼ avocado

  1 6-inch whole-wheat tortilla

  2 tablespoons chimichurri sauce

  Make your own chimichurri sauce by combining 2 tablespoons fresh chopped cilantro, 2 tablespoons Italian parsley, ¼ cup red wine vinegar, ½ diced jalapeño, ¼ cup lemon juice, pinch (⅛ teaspoon) salt and black pepper to taste
- 1 cup Jicama and Red Pepper Slaw (page 228)

Dessert

- ¾ cup frozen strawberry nonfat yogurt

DAY 9

Breakfast

- 1 cup oatmeal cooked with nonfat milk or soymilk, topped with ¼ cup pineapple, ¼ cup mango, and 1 tablespoon chopped walnuts
- 1 cup tea or coffee with 1 tablespoon nonfat milk or soymilk and 1 packet of sugar substitute

Midmorning Snack

- 1-ounce serving of baked potato chips (a good brand is Kettle Crisps) with 2 tablespoons Hummus Dip (page 227)

Lunch

- 1 cup Black Bean Soup (page 194)
- 1 veggie burger with 1 tablespoon Barbecue Sauce (page 188), wrapped in a 6-inch low-sodium whole-wheat tortilla
- 1 nectarine, plum, or tangerine

Midafternoon Snack

- 2 cups air-popped popcorn with pinch (⅛ teaspoon) salt
- 1 apple

Dinner

- 1 cup Tomato Saffron Soup with Orange Essence (page 203)
- 2 cups mixed greens with ½ cup shredded carrots and 2 tablespoons Honey Mustard Dressing (page 184)
- One 4-ounce serving of Spinach-Stuffed Salmon with Mango Sauce (page 222) cooked in ½ teaspoon canola oil and served with ½ cup cooked brown basmati rice

Dessert

- 4 to 6 ounces chocolate pudding (A good ready-made brand choice is sugar-free Jell-O Cups.)

DAY 10

Breakfast

- 1 apple oatmeal pancake
  Mix ¼ cup chopped apple and ¼ cup cooked oatmeal with ¼ to ½ cup whole-grain pancake mix.
- 1 slice low-sodium whole-grain toast with 1 teaspoon 100% fruit spread
- 1 cup tea or coffee with 1 tablespoon nonfat milk or soymilk and 1 packet sugar substitute
- ½ cup fresh blueberries

Midmorning Snack

- 1 cup Cabbage Salad with Coriander and Lemon (see page 229)

Lunch

- 1 baked potato with ½ cup vegetarian chili (Try a canned, low-sodium chili such as Health Valley.)
- 1 cup pico de gallo
- 1 cup cantaloupe

Midafternoon Snack

- 1 cup Chickpea Crunchies
  Toss 1 cup of blotted-dry, cooked chickpeas (garbanzo beans) with ½ teaspoon each of black pepper, cumin, coriander, and cayenne. Spread on a nonstick baking sheet and bake at 400°F until golden brown, about 40 minutes.

Dinner

- 2 sliced tomatoes and 1 cup sliced cucumber with 2 tablespoons aged balsamic vinegar and 1½ teaspoons canola oil

- 1 cup Butternut Squash Soup (page 195)
- 3.5 ounces Elk Chops with Garlic and Sage Crust (page 210) with 1 cup sugar snap peas and ½ cup cooked brown rice

Dessert

- 1 cup fresh melon slices
- 1 cup nonfat plain or no-sugar-added yogurt

DAY 11

Breakfast

- 1 cup fresh fruit
- 1 cup nonfat plain or no-sugar-added yogurt
- Hash browns
  Stir-fry 1 cup diced baked potatoes in a little nonstick cooking spray with onions, paprika, and black pepper until brown.
- 1 cup tea or coffee with 1 tablespoon nonfat milk or soymilk and 1 packet of sugar substitute

Midmorning Snack

- ½ cup carrots, ½ cup celery, with ½ cup red bean dip
  To make dip, combine a can of no-salt-added red beans with ½ cup nonfat yogurt, diced jalapeño to taste, and ½ tablespoon Italian parsley.

Lunch

- 2 cups mixed greens salad topped with 2 tablespoons shrimp-cocktail-style dressing (Blend 1 teaspoon of horseradish with 2 tablespoons of no-salt-added ketchup, such as Westbrae brand.)
- 1 burrito
  One 6-inch whole-grain tortilla
  1 cup grilled veggies
  ½ cup beans, no-salt-added variety
- ½ cup raspberries

Midafternoon Snack

- ½ cup low-fat cottage cheese with ½ cup fresh fruit

Dinner

- 1½ cups iceberg lettuce and ½ cup radicchio with 2 tablespoons vinegar, 1½ teaspoons walnut oil, and black pepper to taste
- 1 cup Tomato Saffron Soup with Orange Essence (page 203)
- 4 ounces Pan-Roasted Lemon Ginger Salmon (page 216), 1 cup snow peas, and ½ cup cooked brown rice with 2 teaspoons low-sodium soy sauce to taste

Dessert

- ½ cup Tia Maria Parfait (page 245)

DAY 12

Breakfast

- 1 cup oatmeal or other hot cereal (cooked with nonfat milk or soymilk) with ½ banana and 2 tablespoons chopped unsalted walnuts
- 1 cup tea or coffee with 1 tablespoon nonfat milk or soymilk and 1 packet sugar substitute

Midmorning Snack

- 1 cup carrot sticks with ½ cup Raita (page 185)

Lunch

- 1 Portobello mushroom burger with 1 tablespoon no-salt-added ketchup, onions and ¼ avocado on whole-wheat bun
- 2 cups mixed greens dressed with 2 tablespoons flavored vinegar and 1 teaspoon low-fat Parmesan cheese

Midafternoon Snack

- 1 cup of grapes
- 1 cup nonfat plain or no-sugar-added yogurt

Dinner

- 2 cups baby spinach with 2 tablespoons Champagne Vinaigrette (page 182)
- 1 cup White Bean Soup
  Combine canned white beans, vegetables, no-salt-added vegetable stock, and chopped fresh parsley. Season with no-salt-added Italian blend seasonings and 1 tablespoon low-sodium soy sauce.
- 1 serving Seafood Romanesco Style (page 218) with ½ cup cooked quinoa.
- 1 cup steamed asparagus

Dessert

- ½ cup fruit sorbet (no sugar added)

DAY 13

Breakfast

- 3-egg-white omelet with:
  ¼ cup tomatoes
  ¼ cup artichokes
  ½ cup mushrooms
- 1 slice low-sodium whole-grain toast with 1 teaspoon 100% fruit spread
- 1 cup tea or coffee with 1 tablespoon nonfat milk or soymilk and 1 packet sugar substitute

Midmorning Snack

- One 6-inch whole-wheat tortilla with ¼ cup salsa mixed with ½ cup corn kernels and 2 tablespoons nonfat sour cream

Lunch

- 1 cup black bean soup
- 3 ounces low-sodium tuna with 1 teaspoon nonfat mayonnaise, 1 tablespoon chopped onion, 1 tablespoon chopped celery, and ¼ avocado on ½ low-sodium whole-wheat bagel
- 1 cup zucchini slices

MID-AFTERNOON SNACK

- 1 pear
- 1 cup nonfat plain or no-sugar-added yogurt

Dinner

- 2 cups mixed greens and ½ cup cherry tomatoes with 1 tablespoon Dijon mustard, 1 tablespoon balsamic vinegar, and 1½ teaspoon canola oil
- 1 cup Butternut Squash Soup (page 195)

- 1 serving Meatless Meatballs (page 215) with 1 cup no-salt-added tomato sauce served over 1 cup cooked whole-wheat pasta

Dessert

- 1 cup fresh cherries

DAY 14

Breakfast

- 1 cup oatmeal or other hot cereal cooked with nonfat milk or soymilk
- 2 tablespoons walnuts
- 1 peach
- 1 cup tea or coffee with 1 tablespoon nonfat milk or soymilk and 1 packet of sugar substitute

Midmorning Snack

- 12 baked tortilla chips
- ½ cup Black Bean Salsa
  Combine ¼ cup black beans, no salt added and ¼ cup salsa, no salt added

Lunch

- 2 cups mixed greens with 2 tablespoons red wine vinegar and 1½ teaspoon canola oil
- 1 cup Tomato and Mushroom Rigatoni
  Use bottled, ready-made marinara sauces (good low-sodium choices are Enrico's, Walnut Acres, and Roselli's) and add your own stir-fried mushrooms, or combine no-salt-added tomato sauce, fresh tomatoes, chopped garlic, and assorted sliced mushrooms. Bring to a boil and simmer for about 15 minutes. Finish by adding freshly chopped basil. Serve on 1 cup cooked whole-wheat pasta.

Midafternoon Snack

- 1 cup watermelon cubes

Dinner

- 2 cups spinach salad with 2 tablespoons aged balsamic vinegar
- 1 cup Black Bean Soup (page 194)
- 4 ounces Seared Whitefish with Rum and Thyme (page 220) with 1 cup cooked quinoa and 1 tablespoon low-sodium soy sauce to taste

Dessert

- Smoothie made with 1 cup nonfat yogurt and ½ cup fresh fruit

PART FIVE

Frequently Asked Questions

HOW CAN I DINE OUT PRITIKIN-STYLE?

Eating Pritikin-style is not about sacrifice; quite the opposite! Our guests are trained to dine out without sacrificing their health or their waistlines. Truly, it isn't difficult. Here are some suggestions for what to eat when dining out.

American/Continental Food

Surprisingly, one of the easiest places to eat Pritikin-style is a good old American steakhouse. Many steakhouses have nice, big salad bars with plenty of fresh veggie and whole bean (such as garbanzo or kidney) choices, as well as great entrée selections like grilled seafood and chicken breasts that aren't smothered with salty, fatty sauces. Steer clear, of course, of the 16-ounce steaks, and run screaming from the 64-ounce ones—even if you get a free television for finishing them. As far as specialty restaurants like the Cheesecake Factory, you can eat healthfully there as well (though one portion of anything at Cheesecake Factory is usually enough to feed at least two people). We take guests at Pritikin to eat there, but if you're tempted the minute you walk in by all those rich, gooey desserts in the glass case, it's best not to walk in at all. One slice of their original cheesecake has 31 grams of saturated fat—more than most of us should have in three days!

Don't ever be shy about asking for substitutions. Even if the menu says your platter comes with fries and mayo-rich coleslaw, many restaurants will happily serve you healthier sides like a baked potato, green salad, corn on the cob, and vegetables.

Here are some suggestions of what you can order.

Appetizer/First Course

- Salad bar: raw vegetables, kidney beans, garbanzo beans, low-cal dressing or vinegar with a touch of oil
- Shrimp cocktail
- Steamed mussels with white wine and garlic
- Brothy soup. Avoid selections with cream and cheese. (Caution: All will likely be high in sodium, so enjoy sparingly.)
- Watch out for rootin'-tootin' specialties like fried whole onions (Outback's Bloomin' Onion has 1,690 calories and 44 grams of fat, and that's *without* the dipping sauce) and stuffed potato skins. An eight-skin order of these cheese-and-bacon–topped babies can easily be the equivalent of swallowing eight strips of bacon, eight tablespoons of sour cream, *and* eight pats of butter.

Entrée

- Grilled or broiled seafood
- Grilled or broiled chicken breast (For both seafood and poultry, ask that your entrée be oil-free or brushed very lightly—not bathed—in oil)
- Steamed lobster
- Petite filet mignon
- More and more restaurants are also serving wild game like bison (buffalo), elk, and moose, which are great choices because they're low in saturated fat—even lower than skinless white poultry.
- Veggie burgers
- Fresh turkey breast sandwich with lettuce, tomato, and mustard

Side

- Steamed or roasted vegetables. Often in American-style restaurants, a side of vegetables is really more like a garnish—a carrot, a forkful of squash, a slice of zucchini. When ordering, ask for three or four times the restaurant's normal serving of vegetables, and say that you'll pay extra. I've never been charged, and I've never been disappointed.

- Corn on the cob—no butter
- Baked potato. Tasty, healthy toppings include salsa, mustard, red pepper flakes, fat-free sour cream, broccoli, and fat-free cheese.
- Baked sweet potato
- Roasted or boiled potatoes, such as red or Yukon gold
- Green beans (ask for flavorings other than butter, such as roasted garlic)

Dessert

- Fruit. Fill up a plate of your favorites from the salad bar. Many often have fresh cut-up selections like pineapple, watermelon, and honeydew.
- Fruit and yogurt parfait
- Sorbet or nonfat ice cream

Chinese Food

Much of Chinese food is sautéed in calorie-dense oil, but you can ask for steamed brown rice and vegetables stir-fried in a small amount of wine or broth instead. Also, request that your dishes be prepared with no added salt, sugar, oil, or soy sauce. Chinese food has several great flavorings available to spice up your food, such as hot mustard, garlic, and ginger.

Another way to ensure that you're not wasting calories is to ask for the sauce that normally accompanies the dish on the side. Then you can still enjoy the flavor by dipping your fork in the sauce before taking a bite of the meal—you'll get all the flavor and a fraction of the calories, fat, and salt.

Appetizer

- Cucumber salad

Rice

- Plain steamed brown rice

Entrée

- Moo Goo Gai Pan (fresh mushrooms with sliced chicken)
- Buddha's Delight (savory vegetarian stew)
- Vegetable lo mein
- Vegetarian or chicken chop suey
- Bean or rice threads or noodle dishes prepared with chicken or tofu
- Broccoli with scallops or chicken
- Whole steamed fish with ginger and garlic (don't eat the skin)

Dessert

- Fresh fruit
- Avoid almond and fortune cookies. Both contain saturated fat and egg yolk.

French Food

When ordering, be sure to tell the waiter you want no added cheese, eggs, butter, or heavy cream-based sauces. Ask that the chef use a minimal amount of oil or none at all, especially if you're trying to lose weight. The same sauce-on-the-side trick where you dip your fork into the sauce and then eat the food is always a good alternative.

Appetizer

- Vegetables vinaigrette
- Grilled vegetables
- Fresh asparagus
- Steamed artichokes (For a tangy, delicious dipping sauce, mix balsamic vinegar with Dijon mustard.)

Soup (Caution: All will be high in sodium, so enjoy sparingly.)

- Onion soup (without cheese)
- Consommé
- Lentil soup

Salad
- Salads of steamed or marinated fresh vegetables
- Salad Niçoise without oil or egg yolk

Entrée
- Roasted chicken
- Grilled chicken or fish
- Poached salmon
- Fish stew (bouillabaisse)
- Filet mignon

Indian Food

Typically, southern Indian food is quite spicy, while much of northern Indian cuisine is made with cream. Request no cream or other saturated-fat-rich or calorie-rich ingredients, such as ghee (clarified butter), coconut, and oil. Also, request no added salt and sugar.

Appetizer
- Papadum (baked lentil wafers typically made with oil, so go easy if you're trying to lose weight)

Soup
- Samber (vegetarian)
- Mulligatawny (lentil and vegetables)
- Dhal Rasam (lentil and peppers)

Salad
- Chopped salad with onion, tomatoes, and lettuce

Bread
Typically, these breads are oiled after they are baked, so to avoid the extra calories, request that they serve you the bread directly from the oven.

- Chapati (whole wheat)
- Nan (poppyseed)
- Kuicha (leavened baked bread)

Entrée

- Chicken Tandoori
- Chicken Tikka (roasted with mild spices)
- Chicken Saag (cooked with spinach—ask the chef to hold the cream)
- Chicken Vindaloo (very spicy dish cooked with potato)
- Shrimp Bhuna (cooked with vegetables)
- Vegetable Biryani (basmati rice with vegetables)
- Aloo-Gobi (cauliflower and potato)
- Pullao (basmati rice)
- Chana dishes (delicious preparations made with garbanzo beans)

Dessert

- Fresh fruit

Italian Food

It can be very easy to get a delicious and healthy meal at an Italian restaurant. Ask that the chef use only a minimum amount of oil, or none at all, and request dishes with no added salt. Insist on no added butter or cheese. Remember, even a few shakes of cheese add saturated fat and a whole lot of calories!

Appetizer

- Steamed mussels or clams
- Grilled vegetables
- Steamed artichokes

Salad

- Salad with no meat, cheese, or olives. For a dressing, use vinegar or lemon juice.
- Arugula with balsamic vinegar—a simple yet very elegant and flavorful salad

Soup

- Minestrone is a possible choice. Most varieties have only small amounts of oil, but the salt content will be high, so avoid it if you have hypertension.

Pasta

- Ask for whole-wheat pasta. If it isn't available, white pasta without egg is the next best choice. Be aware that fresh "homemade" pasta may contain some egg. Avoid stuffed pastas such as ravioli and tortellini.
- Order a meatless tomato sauce, such as marinara or pomodoro. If the sauce contains oil and salt, use it sparingly.
- A creative and delicious alternative: Request fresh, chopped tomatoes, basil, garlic, and a splash of balsamic vinegar.
- Another option: Order a side of grilled or steamed vegetables and mix them with your pasta.

Entrée

- There is hidden calorie-dense fat (usually oil and butter) in many Italian entrées such as chicken Marsala. Play it safe and order simple grilled fish or chicken, or pasta primavera.

Vegetable

- Order vegetables without butter or sauce.

Dessert

- Fruit salad
- Fresh strawberries in Marsala wine

Japanese Food

Having sushi is an excellent way to dine out Pritikin-style—and one of my favorites. A healthy alternative to soy sauce is lemon juice or, for something a little zestier, try rice wine vinegar or small amounts (a teaspoon) of low-sodium soy souce. When possible, ask for sushi rolls to be prepared with brown rather than white rice. For cooked Japanese dishes, request no added salt, sugar, or oils; you can add wasabi for added spice. Avoid the deep-fried tempura dishes.

Appetizer
- Cucumber salad in vinaigrette
- Grilled vegetables
- Edamame (steamed soybeans), without the salt sprinkled on top

Soup
- Miso soup (though beware: it is high in sodium, so enjoy sparingly)

Rice
- Steamed brown rice

Entrée
- Seafood Sunomono (with vegetables and vinegar)
- Sushi
- Sashimi
- Sukiyaki
- Mizutaki (chicken and vegetables simmered in water)
- Fish that is steamed, grilled, or roasted

Dessert
- Fresh fruit

Mexican Food

Mexican food offers some healthy options, but you need to order carefully. For your heart's sake, request no lard, sour cream, cheese, fried pastry, or fried taco shells. For your waistline, request no oil and just small amounts of guacamole or sliced avocado for your salad. The rice and beans in Mexican restaurants may be pre-cooked with either oil or lard; you can always call ahead to find out. If only a little oil has been used, don't be too concerned, but do avoid restaurants that use lard.

Appetizer
- Ask the waiter to bring steamed corn tortillas (rather than fried chips) with the salsa.

Soup
Both of these choices are healthful as well as tasty, but be aware that sodium content will probably be high.
- Black bean
- Gazpacho

Entrée
- Chicken fajitas, sautéed with minimal or no oil to avoid the extra calories, with steamed corn tortillas
- Soft, steamed tostada with beans, salsa, lettuce, onion, and shredded vegetables
- Chicken enchilada (no cheese)
- Soft chicken or fish taco (no cheese). Ask for no breading or dressing on the fish.
- Seafood Veracruz
- Chicken or seafood taco salad (without the taco shells)
- Arroz con pollo (rice with chicken)

Bread
- Steamed corn tortillas

Thai Food

In most restaurants, curry dishes have coconut milk as a base, so check before you order. Ask that vegetables be stir-fried in a small amount of broth or wine, or a minimum of oil. Request no salt or calorie-dense nuts, and avoid heart-harmful coconut milk and lard.

Appetizer
- Satay (marinated grilled beef or chicken). Avoid the peanut dipping sauce.
- Steamed mussels
- Thai garden salad
- Steamed rice
- Seafood kebob

Soup
- Crystal noodle soup
- Talay Thong (seafood, beans, and vegetables)

Entrée
- Thai chicken (hold the cashews if you're trying to lose weight)
- Sweet and sour chicken (which will probably contain sugar)
- Poy Siam (sautéed seafood)
- Scallops/bamboo shoots/vegetable boat
- Pad Thai (vegetables and spices)

Dessert
- Fresh fruit

WHAT DO FOOD LABELS MEAN?

Trying to make sense out of food labels is like trying to sleep at a rock concert. The best intentions can have disastrous results. A lot of Americans tried in the 1990s to cut back on fatty, calorie-dense foods, and government statistics show that we did eat less fat as a percentage of our total calories. The problem is that we are now eating more calories overall, so the *total amount of fat* we're eating is higher than ever.

How did this happen? Food labels are in part to blame. Despite good intentions, many of us have no idea what we're eating because we can't make sense of the labels. Few people understand the role food manufacturers—and legal but misleading and deceptive marketing—have played in this. Unrealistic government regulations and deceptive practices by the food industry are so complex and confusing that we're often buying junk when we think we're buying good, healthy food. Products marketed as low fat could be 40, 50, or even 70 percent fat. Products marketed as fat free could be 100 percent fat. And now, "trans fat free products" can contain small amounts of trans fats. While most Americans surveyed say they read labels to try and pick healthier foods, few, if any, have actually figured out how to use the labels or understand the marketing of food.

One of the most popular lectures at the Pritikin Center is the one we give on how to read food labels. It seems that *everyone* wants to learn to decipher the confusing numbers and jargon on common packaging! On the next few pages you'll see just how confusing and misleading food labels can be (and why), and you'll get the knowledge and power you need to make better choices when buying foods.

Misleading Information

Ann is a 42-year-old secretary at my hospital. She has struggled with her weight throughout her life. One day I saw Ann spraying a cooking spray on a slice of toast she had heated up in the toaster. Intrigued, I asked her why. She pointed to the front label boldly stating "naturally fat free" and the nutrition box stating "0 calories" and "0 fat." She was spraying it on anything and everything. It tasted good, and better yet, "didn't have any calories." Was she right?

If you're trying to lose weight, cooking spray certainly looks like the way to do it. The label boldly announces that it's "fat free," and the nutrition box says it has 0 calories and 0 grams of fat. Wow, it looks as if you could use the cooking spray on everything and not add a single calorie to your diet. Plus, says the label, it's "all natural." Let's take a closer look.

FAT-FREE OLIVE OIL SPRAY

Nutrition Facts

Serving Size	About ⅓ Second Spray (.266g)
Servings Per Container	About 438
Calories	0
Calories from Fat	0
Total Fat	0g
Saturated Fat	0g
Cholesterol	0mg
Sodium	0mg
Total Carbohydrate	0g
Protein	0g

INGREDIENTS:

100% imported olive oil, grain alcohol from corn (added for clarity), lethicin from soybeans, propellant

Under the ingredient list, the first, and therefore main, ingredient is olive oil. Olive oil is 100 percent fat. Pure fat. So how does a product that's 100 percent fat get sold to us a "fat free" product? Let's take a look at the Nutrition Facts box. The serving size is .266 grams (¼ of a gram), which adds up to about one-third of a second of spray. The manufacturer can call that serving "0 grams" of fat and "0 calories" because our government allows any serving that's less than one-half gram, no matter what the ingredients are, to be rounded down to zero.

But who's spraying their skillet for a "don't-blink-or-you'll-miss-it" third of a second? As a cardiologist, I know that one-third of a second is pretty short, just about the time between your heart's lub and its dub. The fact is, most of us coat our toast or skillets for a good five to six seconds, and those few seconds add up to about 50 calories. Ounce for ounce, cooking spray contains as many calories as butter. Bottom line:

cooking spray, a product that is virtually all fat, is being sold to us as one that's "fat free." Are you mad? I sure am!

Want to get even madder? Consider this one. Bite-sized "healthy" brand ice-cream sandwiches, by the claims on the front of the package, look like the healthiest thing ever. They have no butterfat, they're lactose free, they're only 130 calories per serving, and if you eat enough of them, you may even get as trim and fit as the two racing bicyclists at the top of the box. Now we'll check the Nutrition Facts box and ingredients list:

ICE-CREAM SANDWICH

Nutrition Facts

Serving Size	1 sandwich (40 grams)
Servings Per Container	8
Calories	130
Calories from Fat	54
Total Fat	6g
Saturated Fat	1g
Trans Fat	0g
Total Carbs	17g
Fiber	0g
Sugars	9g
Protein	2g
Butterfat	0g
Lactose	0g
Cholesterol	0g
Sodium	121mg

INGREDIENTS

Water, sugar, corn syrup solids, contains one or more of the following oils (corn, soy, coconut, and palm), soy protein, tofu, cocoa butter, vanilla, soy lecithin, guar seed gum, carageenan, carob bean gum, salt.

Chocolate Wafer: Unbleached wheat flour, sugar, caramel color, soybean oil, yellow corn flour, cocoa, modified corn starch, salt, baking soda, vegetable mono and diglycerides, soy lecithin.

The Nutrition Facts box and ingredient list reveal what's really in these desserts. First of all, they're little; one serving size is tiny. One serving, or sandwich, is 40 grams, which adds up to 1.4 ounces, or one quick mouthful. So you're probably eating at least two, which means you're swallowing a hefty 260 calories in about 20 seconds.

And what's in these "no butterfat" calories? For starters, a lot of fat. A 130-calorie serving gets 54 of its calories from fat. That means that 42 percent of its calories are pure fat.

The ingredient list doesn't look healthy either. Two of the first three ingredients in the ice-cream filling (sugar and corn syrup solids) are refined sugars, so this product is loaded with sugar. In the filling you'll also find artery-clogging saturated fat in the form of cocoa butter. Yes, a product advertised as having "no butterfat" still has lots of saturated fat.

It gets worse. You'd think that an ice-cream sandwich sold in health food stores would use whole grains for its wafers, but the first ingredient is "unbleached wheat flour," which sounds healthy but is just plain old white flour. And guess how these wafers got their wholesome brown color? Ingredient 3—the caramel color. That's browned sugar. Why even bother traveling to a health food store? More than 95 percent of the calories in this product are refined sugars, refined grains, and refined fats and oils. With zero fiber and as much salt as potato chips, this product has more than 1,400 calories per pound, giving it a high calorie density. Not exactly a "health" food, is it?

Don't despair! The enemies of healthy eating need not defeat you. With a little detective work and some simple but very important rules, you will avoid the confusion, see through the deception, and discover the truly healthy food in your market.

When it comes to deciphering food labels, there are three key things you need to remember:

- Never, ever believe the health claims on the front of the package,
- Always check the Nutrition Facts box, and
- Always check the ingredients list.

The Nutrition Facts Box

On every package, there is a Nutrition Facts box. Within that box, you'll want to focus on the following listings:

- serving size
- number of servings per package
- calories per serving
- calories from fat
- saturated and trans fat grams in the serving
- sodium (mg) in the serving

Serving size

Though the government standardized most serving sizes years ago, many products still post unrealistically small sizes, like that "⅓ second of oil spray." That's about 120th of an ounce—far less than most people could, or would, spray on a pan with even just one tiny squirt.

Number of servings per package

Decades ago, many products were in fact single servings. A bottle of cola was one serving. One small candy bar was one serving. Today, many products are "super-sized" and contain multiple servings. Be realistic. Are you really going to drink only eight ounces of that 20-ounce beverage, or eat only half of that bagel? A 20-ounce bottle of cola contains 2.5 servings, at 110 calories each. Invariably, all 275 calories go down. Is it any surprise that many of us are super-sized ourselves?

Calories per serving

Watch out for foods that pack a lot of calories per serving. Calorie-dense foods put on the pounds without filling you up (remember, foods that are calorie-light are less than 500 calories per pound).

Sometimes food manufacturers pack their products with calories but announce they're "reduced in carbs" or "reduced in fat" and are therefore just what you need if you're trying to lose weight. They're just what you *don't* need. Here's one example:

As the name suggests, Carb Fit tortilla chips, popular during the low-carb craze a few years ago, were marketed to people longing to be fit. The front of the package told us they were "all natural," made of soy and corn, and best of all, had only five grams of "net carbs" (whatever those are). But let's compare the Nutrition Facts of Carb Fit Tortilla Chips with the Nutrition Facts of Doritos.

Carb Fit Tortilla Chips	Doritos
Serving size for both is 1 ounce (about 11 chips)	
Nutrition Facts	Nutrition Facts
Calories: 150	Calories: 140
Calories from Fat: 80	Calories from Fat: 70
Total Fat: 8g	Total Fat: 8g
Cholesterol: 0mg	Cholesterol: 0mg
Sodium: 280mg	Sodium: 180mg
Total Carbohydrate: 9g	Total Carbohydrate: 17g
Fiber: 4g	Fiber: 1g
Sugar: 0g	Sugar: 1g
Protein: 9g	Protein: 2g

What's the difference if you're trying to lose weight? Both are packed with calories.

In fact, Carb Fit chips have *more* calories per serving than Doritos. With 150 calories packed into one small one-ounce serving, you can virtually feel your pants ripping at the seams as you rip open one bag after another. Chances are you will, because they're marketed as "low-carb" and "good for you." Both Carb Fit and Doritos can easily put on weight. Both are calorie-dense junk foods.

Calories from fat

Try to keep the fat calories less than about 20 percent of the total calories for processed food and less than about 30 percent for meat and poultry. The percentage of fat calories in seafood can exceed 30 percent because it is generally high in essential omega-3 fats. Don't be fooled by all those 93%, 98%, and 99% fat-free claims. Here's one that fools just about everyone.

Did you know that "2% fat" milk actually gets about 35 percent of its calories from fat? How does the dairy industry get away with this? The government allows it to measure fat as a percentage *by weight*. By weight, the fat in milk doesn't add up to much, just 2 percent of the total liquid weight. But here's the problem: There's never been a health guideline that has told us to watch fat by percentage of weight. Health experts have always directed us to watch fat by *percentage of calories*. A one-cup serving of this milk (see Nutrition Facts box below) has 130 calories, and 45 of those are fat calories. So this milk is actually about 35 percent fat. That's right, more than one-third of its calories come from fat, and three-fifths of that fat is deadly saturated fat.

2% REDUCED FAT MILK
Nutrition Facts

Serving Size	1 cup (236mL)

Amount per Serving

Calories	130
Calories from Fat	45
Total Fat	5g
Saturated Fat	3g
Trans Fat	0g
Cholesterol	20mg
Sodium	125mg
Total Carbohydrate	13g
Fiber	0g
Sugar	12g
Protein	8g

In "99% fat-free" soup, the fat may be as much as 77 percent of total calories. At the meat counter, the lean ground meat may be labeled

93 percent fat-free by weight, but the fat equals 46 percent of the calories. Legally speaking, this may be truth in advertising, but it is also deceptive and misleading. Congressman Christopher Shays seemed to agree strongly with me about how misleading these practices are when I spoke on a food panel arranged by one of the brilliant deans at Yale's School of Management, Dr. Jeffrey Sonnenfeld. One hopes that Congress will do something to stop these misleading practices.

Saturated and trans fat grams in the serving

Saturated fats should be limited to fewer than five to ten grams or 5 percent of calories consumed per day total, so you're best off selecting processed foods with not more than one or two grams. Do not eat foods listing any amount of trans fat. Foods still may contain less than one-half gram per serving and be listed as having zero grams of trans fat or saturated fat, but this deception can often be unmasked by looking at the ingredients.

Sodium (mg) in the serving

Our bodies need fewer than 300 milligrams of sodium a day. Fewer than 1,500 milligrams of sodium per day is recommended by the Institute of Medicine. We Americans eat an average 3,500 to 5,000 milligrams daily. Since it's very difficult to keep track of calories, calorie density, and sodium, here is an easy solution. Keep the sodium in milligrams fewer than the calories. If, for example, the calories are 200, the sodium should be fewer than 200. Assuming you're sticking to a Pritikin-style diet, your sodium intake will be limited to about 2,000 milligrams per day if it doesn't exceed your calorie intake. It will probably be even less, as it is at the Pritikin Center, because you'll be eating many of your calories from fruits and vegetables.

Surprisingly, the leading contributors of salt in the American diet are bread products. Many breads and other grain-based foods, such as pretzels and cornflakes, contain more salt, ounce for ounce, than potato chips and French fries. That doesn't mean chips and fries are good for you; it just means that you need to watch out for the amount of sodium in bread products.

It's shocking how much sodium there is in some "reduced sodium" products. Progresso's new "Healthy Favorites" canned soups, for example, proudly proclaim they have "50% less sodium." The sodium in one serving is 470 milligrams, a tolerable amount if this is your entire lunch. But one serving is just half a can, and most of us cannot make a meal of half a can of chicken noodle soup. The whole can contains 940 milligrams of sodium, *more than half the sodium we should have in one day.*

The Ingredient List

When you turn your eye to the ingredient list, there are three main things for which you want to be scouring:

1. Avoid added sugars in the first three to five ingredients.
2. Avoid all hydrogenated and tropical oils and saturated fats.
3. Select unrefined whole grains.

Avoid added sugars

Ingredients are listed in descending order of weight, the heaviest being the first, second heaviest the second, and so on. So if sugar is listed as the first ingredient, there's more sugar than anything else in the product. Sugar may be listed as such or it may be masked as corn syrup, sorghum, rice or maple syrup, molasses, honey, malted barley, barley malt, sorbitol, dextrose, glucose, or fructose.

Whole fruit as an ingredient, even if it is a sweet fruit, is okay, but added fruit juice, such as grape juice concentrate (really just another name for sugar), should be avoided. The lower down the list you see sugar, the better. And if you see several kinds of sugar anywhere on the list, chances are the total amount of sugar is excessive.

Avoid all hydrogenated oils and tropical oils and saturated fats

Steer clear of all hydrogenated oils, which may contain trans fat, even if not listed as such. Avoid all tropical oils, such as palm, palm kernel, and coconut oil, which may be disguised as healthy-sounding vegetable oil. And as much as possible, choose foods with no saturated fats. Ingredients such as lard, butter, coconut, cocoa butter, shortening, margarine, chocolate, chicken fat, cheese, and whole and part-skim dairy products are high in saturated fat. Avoid other cholesterol-raising ingredients, too, including eggs, egg yolks, tallow, suet, and schmaltz.

Select unrefined *whole* grains

There are a lot of fancy names today for breads and the grains they use, like seven-grain and multi-grain. But those seven grains could be seven white flours! Have you ever seen anything healthier-looking than the front label of Pepperidge Farm Light Style Seven Grain Bread? It's "light," it has "no trans fat," and it has seven grains. Maybe those grains are even ground in a little country barn like the one on the label. But all these grains are refined white grains, starting with the first—unbromated unbleached enriched wheat flour. That may sound healthy, but it's *not* a whole-grain flour.

Buy bread, pastas, and other grain products that show as their first ingredient *whole* grain, such as whole-wheat flour or sprouted whole-grain kernels. Don't be fooled by healthy-sounding names like wheat flour, enriched flour, multi-grain flour, semolina flour, durum flour, unbleached flour, bleached flour, or even spinach flour. These are all *refined* white flours. It's got to say "whole." Look for at least three grams of fiber per serving, which usually means the product is mostly, if not all, whole grain.

Should every food you select meet these criteria? That's certainly the Pritikin gold standard, but it's a lofty goal. It is possible to achieve if you eat out often, but much easier if you prepare your own food. That would actually involve buying food in the produce section of your supermarket and learning how to use those antiquated devices in the kitchen, such as pots, pans, and stoves. (A warning for the inexperienced: unlike microwave ovens, stove gets hot!) Though healthy eating doesn't always require pots and pans; even the most kitchen-challenged among us can peel a banana, rinse strawberries, and break open a bag of baby carrots.

If you prepare all your own food, fine. If not, the reality is that food that doesn't meet the Pritikin guidelines should be kept to a minimum and balanced by more really healthy food.

CAN I EAT CHOCOLATE?

How about those forbidden foods, such as bacon, cheese, ribs, and "death-by-chocolate" desserts? Can you eat them?

Go ahead and enjoy them—*sparingly*. I do, and I weigh 140 pounds. Though such foods are not recommended by the Pritikin or any legitimate health program, nobody can bat 1,000 all the time!

Michael, whom you met in Chapter 3, is a Pritikin success story. He has lost and kept off 80 pounds. Almost every day he eats Pritikin style. But seven days out of the year—his birthday, Thanksgiving, Christmas, the Fourth of July, and his daughters' and wife's birthdays—he allows himself to eat whatever he wants, from bacon to beignets. He enjoys himself, then goes back to enjoying the Pritikin Program.

The problem with the American diet is not the occasional tasty bonbon or six-ounce juicy steak, but a steady diet of cheeseburgers, fries, and colas, full of saturated fat, salt, and sugar and devoid of fruits, vegetables, essential oils, fiber, and vitamins. At one time our government actually considered ketchup a vegetable. If you put five packets of ketchup on a hamburger, you met your daily requirement of vegetables. We do not have a heritage of enlightened nutrition. Our food industry certainly doesn't, either.

If you are one of those people who consider chocolate to be an essential food group, go ahead and enjoy it once in a while. There is little question that chocolate is an emotional reward as well as a tasty treat. Some data suggest that chocolate releases endorphins, which are intrinsic mood elevators. The effect is especially evident in women, many of whom with good judgment prefer chocolate to men.

Interestingly, chocolate is a good example of how complex food can be. Cocoa powder, the basis for chocolate, is rich in complex antioxidant chemicals that increase nitric oxide and decrease blood pressure. Unfortunately, cocoa powder is mixed with milk fat to make milk chocolate, thus introducing considerable amounts of saturated fat. Darker chocolates may be a little better because they lack milk fat, but all chocolate, dark and light, is full of calorie-dense refined sugar, which could certainly derail your weight-loss efforts if you're consuming it regularly.

So, all that to say: indulge sparingly!

HOW CAN I HELP MY CHILD EAT HEALTHIER?

Here are a few suggestions to help your child break away from America's march toward almost universal obesity.

In General

- Be a good role model. Don't preach what you can't practice.
- Limit television viewing, especially of kids' shows. Almost every commercial is for something they shouldn't eat or don't need.
- Never have the TV on during dinner. That time should be reserved for enjoying food and conversing as a family.
- Insist that they eat dinner at home. Kids don't need separate meals. They need to be exposed to good adult food very early in life. Eating well is a habit, just like eating poorly.
- Show them how to shop on-the-go at salad bars and the deli section of supermarkets rather than settling for just-as-expensive fast food.

- Walk to neighborhood restaurants. Kids naturally love physical activity if adequately exposed to it.
- Get involved in your school's lunch program. Don't complain about what your kids eat at school if you are not prepared to do something about it.
- Spoil your kids a little with healthy, tasty treats when they come home from school and while they are doing their homework. Teach them that good eating is not dieting!

Breakfast

- The most satisfying, healthy breakfast is hot oatmeal topped with skim milk and fresh fruit instead of sugar.
- In second place is whole-grain, no-sugar-added cold cereal, also topped with skim milk and fresh fruit. Most kids love berries— strawberries, blueberries, or whatever kind you have on hand to toss on top. If they don't like cereal, try a smoothie made from nonfat strawberry yogurt, orange juice, a ripe banana, and ice.

Lunch

- Almost every child loves peanut butter and jelly sandwiches. Just use whole-grain bread and 100-percent fruit preserve (no added sugar). For variety, substitute a banana for the jelly.
- Pack a school lunch of chili or shredded roast chicken from the night before if your child can keep it cold.
- A hearty soup packed in a thermos with whole-grain crackers makes a wonderful lunch in the winter.

Dinner

- Give kids choices. Line up a buffet of tasty, healthy food. For example, start with whole-grain pitas or corn tortillas. Let your kids stuff them with roasted chicken breast, pinto or black beans, tomatoes, shredded lettuce, sliced avocado, diced onions, and salsa. The Mexican Tortilla Feast is always a hit with the kids at Pritikin.

- Learn how to make and lightly dress big, tasty salads to start out dinner.
- The same goes for soups. They're satisfying and generally low calorie. Just remember to go easy on the salt.
- Whole-grain bread, white and sweet potatoes, and pasta are not the enemy; the mounds of butter, sour cream, bacon bits, cheese, and sausage on top of them are. Teach your children to enjoy starches without these added unhealthy calories.
- Potato chips and French fries are junk food. Instead, make baked potato skins seasoned with garlic or anything except oil. They're about 60 calories per skin if you scoop out most of the inside. See our recipe on page 226.

Snacks

- Make sure that there are healthy snacks around, especially in the afternoon when kids are really hungry.
- Microwave air-popped popcorn, unsalted nuts, and dried fruit make a great trail mix–like snack.
- Mix raw carrots, cauliflower, apple slices, and orange wedges in a ziplock bag and refrigerate.
- Blending a little orange juice and frozen strawberries makes a tasty, low-calorie sorbet.
- Fresh fruit is always a winner. A whole pineapple contains fewer calories (about 200) than a handful of gummy bears.
- Supermarkets usually have single servings of peeled baby carrots ready to eat.
- Flavored nonfat yogurt can become as much of a treat as ice cream.
- Freeze seedless grapes and banana slices.

WHAT DO MY CHOLESTEROL VALUES MEAN?

Cholesterol is a complex molecule found in all animals—including humans. It is circulated in our blood and is found in cell walls and several hormones. Animal life would not exist without cholesterol, but then again, neither would atherosclerosis. Our bodies can manufacture all of the cholesterol we need. We do not need to eat any. The excess from the food we eat, such as meat, cheese, and milk, can do a lot of damage.

The bloodstream is a two-way highway for cholesterol. Although all tissues make cholesterol, the liver makes most of the circulating cholesterol. The liver packages cholesterol along with protein and triglycerides in big, buoyant particles called very low-density lipoprotein, or VLDL. As VLDL circulates in the blood, the light triglyceride molecules are stripped away, changing VLDL to low-density lipoprotein, or LDL. The triglyceride molecules are burned for energy or stored in fat tissues if they are not immediately needed. The cholesterol left in the LDL is distributed to tissues. Any excess LDL gets deposited in the walls of the arteries and injures the endothelium, which then begins the atherosclerotic process. Thus LDL cholesterol is the "bad" cholesterol.

Unlike the liver, the arteries cannot break down excess cholesterol and need to ship it back to the liver, which excretes it into the intestines as part of bile. The cholesterol returning to the liver is carried by a dense, protein-rich lipoprotein called high-density lipoprotein, or HDL. The cholesterol in HDL is therefore "good" cholesterol because it is being shipped back to the liver for excretion. Think of LDL (bad) cholesterol as garbage and HDL (good) cholesterol as the garbage trucks. Refuse piles up if you have too much garbage and/or too few trucks to haul it away.

Total Cholesterol Values

Your cholesterol panel measures your total cholesterol, LDL (bad) cholesterol, HDL (good) cholesterol, and triglycerides. Hundreds of studies have shown that heart disease increases at higher levels of total choles-

terol. The most conservative recommendation for acceptable total cholesterol is lower than 200. This value is very conservative, because more
than one-third of people who get heart disease have values between 150
and 200. Heart disease rarely occurs in people with total cholesterol below 150.

Is there a perfect total cholesterol value? Yes. American men taking part in the Multiple Risk Factor Intervention Trial had the lowest mortality at a total cholesterol value of 122. That's the ideal target
number. If you recall his story at the beginning of this book, Nathan
Pritikin achieved a perfect 120 total cholesterol, and clean coronary
arteries.

A total cholesterol value of 122 sounds very low to most people,
since the average cholesterol in America is 206. In nature, however, cholesterol of 122 is the rule. Human beings are still biologically primates;
like it or not, we still share 99 percent of our genes with chimpanzees. (I
know a few people, including some colleagues, who probably share an
even higher percentage, but that's a whole other topic.) The total cholesterol of primates ranges from 110 to 140. Living in the wild, primates
never develop heart disease. Primitive hunter-gatherers living today
have about the same cholesterol values, and they, too, never develop
heart disease. By every line of evidence, having a total cholesterol value
of or around 122 is the best way to avoid heart disease.

LDL (Bad) Cholesterol

Your LDL (bad) cholesterol measurement is a better gauge of your heart
disease risk than total cholesterol. The National Cholesterol Education
Program teaches that acceptable LDL (bad) cholesterol is less than 130
or 160, depending on other risk factors. This standard also makes no
sense. Most Americans with heart disease have LDL (bad) cholesterol
values below 160, and many even below 130. Three-quarters of heart attack sufferers would not qualify for cholesterol treatment the day before
their coronary episodes based on these standards.

The latest guidelines do acknowledge that a desirable LDL (bad) cholesterol number is now less than 100. More than 20 years before the National Cholesterol Education Program got around to reducing its definition of a "desirable" LDL cholesterol to less than 100, the Pritikin Longevity Center adopted this guideline for the prevention of coronary artery disease. For regression of advanced atherosclerosis, our Pritikin team now recommends LDL (bad) cholesterol be 70 or less. Odds are that in a few years, the National Cholesterol Education Program will recognize that even their "desirable" guideline of 100 is too conservative, and will likely drop it closer to current Pritikin guidelines for regression of heart disease.

Should those of you without heart disease have the same LDL (bad) cholesterol goal? We believe the answer is yes. Admittedly, we do not have the same wealth of data for healthy individuals as we have for those with heart disease. What we do know is that almost every study involving lowering cholesterol has shown a decrease in heart disease and stroke. A recent trial of more than 15,000 volunteers without heart disease found that cardiovascular events decreased when LDL (bad) cholesterol was lowered from about 100 to about 60.

The basic principle of LDL (bad) cholesterol, whether you have heart disease or not, is exactly the same as for golf: in all cases, lower scores win.

HLD (Good) Cholesterol

If LDL (bad) cholesterol is like golf, then HDL (good) cholesterol is basketball: higher scores win. As HDL (good) cholesterol increases (up to a value of about 100), heart disease decreases. Heart disease occurs infrequently at HDL (good) cholesterol values above 60 in men and above 70 in women; these are considered desirable values. By American standards, the minimal acceptable value of HDL (good) cholesterol is 40 for men and 50 for women.

However, if you have little garbage (LDL or bad cholesterol) to begin with, you may not need as many garbage trucks (HDL or good cholesterol). Populations with the lowest rates of heart disease in the world, such as the people living in Okinawa and in other rural regions of Asia, have low levels of HDL (good) cholesterol—often in the 20s and 30s. But their total and LDL (bad) cholesterol levels are very low, too. Colin Campbell of Cornell University, studying rural Chinese, found that their diet consisted largely of vegetables, fruits, rice, and other grains—and three times more fiber than a typical American diet. Their death rate from heart disease was *94 percent lower than* that of American men. In short, while high HDL (good) cholesterol levels are desirable, total and LDL (bad) cholesterol levels that are very low are even more desirable.

Triglycerides

Triglycerides, as the name implies, are three fatty acid molecules tied together. Elevated blood triglycerides occur in metabolic syndrome and predict the development of diabetes.

The National Cholesterol Education Program recommends that triglycerides be reduced below 150, but we believe 100 is a more desirable goal.

If you are concerned about any of your cholesterol numbers, please refer to the next question, which talks about how you can adopt a cholesterol-improving lifestyle.

HOW CAN I IMPROVE MY CHOLESTEROL?

Many people with high cholesterol want to go straight to medications, which are very effective and also have few serious side effects. But by doing so, they will have missed an opportunity to lose weight and look better, become more physically fit and happy, and lessen their risk of cancer, diabetes, high blood pressure, arthritis, and gall bladder disease. All of these conditions can be prevented by the same lifestyle changes that reduce heart disease. They are also spending a lot more money. As you already know, we strongly believe that making healthy lifestyle changes is always better than taking medications.

Ideal Cholesterol Values

- Total: less than 150, ideally 122
- LDL (bad) cholesterol: less than 100, ideally less than 70
- HDL (good) cholesterol: above 60 for men and above 70 for women
- Triglycerides: less than 100

In Part Two of this book, you learned the 10 Pritikin Essentials, all of which contribute to a cholesterol-lowering lifestyle. An analysis of more than 4,500 people who went to the Pritikin Longevity Center found that at the end of three weeks, their total cholesterol had dropped an average of 23 percent. They also saw an average 23 percent drop in LDL (bad) cholesterol, and triglycerides fell 33 percent.

We encourage you to try the lifestyle changes outlined in this book, and summarized below, to improve your cholesterol. Again, if these changes do not improve your cholesterol enough, then absolutely talk to your physician about taking a statin or other cholesterol-lowering drug. Do not hesitate!

Lowering Total and LDL (Bad) Cholesterol

The Pritikin approach to reducing total and LDL (bad) cholesterol is:
- Eat much less saturated and trans fat.
- Eat less cholesterol.
- Lose excess weight.
- Use a stanol- or sterol-fortified supplement or margarine (but go easy on the margarine if you're trying to lose weight—it is very high in calories).
- Eat more food high in soluble fiber. (Remember BYOBB: beans, yams, oats, barley, berries.)
- Increase physical activity.

Increasing HDL (Good) Cholesterol

Increasing HDL (good) cholesterol is more difficult, but not less important, than reducing LDL (bad) cholesterol. The Pritikin approach to increasing HDL (good) cholesterol is:

- Exercise more and regularly.
- Lose excess weight.
- Drink alcohol in moderation (and responsibly).
- Stop smoking.
- Eat fewer trans fats.

In short, take up running from bar to bar. Please note that I did not
say to *drive* from bar to bar. Both running about 10 miles per week and
drinking moderately increase HDL (good) cholesterol 10 to 15 percent.
It is unclear whether you can overdo running, but too much alcohol is
obviously a major health problem. Smoking cessation and avoiding dietary trans fats also increase HDL (good) cholesterol.

Statin and fibrate drugs increase HDL (good) cholesterol modestly,
but niacin increases it 10 to 40 percent, depending on the dose. Niacin
can be bought over the counter, but it is associated with several side effects, some of which are potentially serious. Its use should be discussed
with your physician even if you don't get a prescription.

Lowering Triglycerides

Triglycerides increase with weight and are almost always elevated in diabetes and its cousin, metabolic syndrome. The Pritikin approach to lowering triglycerides is:

- Lose excess weight.
- Eat less sugar and other highly refined and processed carbohydrates.

- Eat more fish and omega-3 fats.
- Drink very little alcohol.
- Increase physical activity.

One episode of exercise can lower triglycerides for up to two days. Eating fish and taking omega-3 supplements (three to five grams of omega-3 fish oil per day, taken in capsule form) also lower triglycerides. Sugars, including alcohol, can dramatically increase triglycerides, as, of course, can fatty foods. In fact, unlike LDL (bad) and HDL (good) cholesterols, which change slowly after eating, triglycerides increase 30 to 100 percent after a single fat-containing meal and can remain elevated for up to eight hours after eating.

Fibrates, niacin, and statins also lower triglycerides, but lifestyle changes are still the most effective means.

AM I AT RISK FOR DIABETES?

If you are overweight or obese, the short answer is yes.

We diagnose diabetes by measuring either fasting blood sugar or blood sugar after a sugar load. Normal fasting blood sugar is below 100, but really desirable fasting sugar is below 85. You have diabetes if your fasting sugar is above 125 and you have borderline diabetes if it is between 100 and 125. You have diabetes if your glucose tolerance test is 200 or above and borderline diabetes if it is 140 to 199.

Diabetes can not only be diagnosed, it can be predicted. Central obesity, which entails a waist circumference greater than 40 inches in a man and 35 inches in a woman, is the best indicator that diabetes is a genuine risk. Assuming that you are not pregnant, stand up straight and look down at your feet. Do not suck in your gut! If your belly blocks your feet from your view, you are well on your way to developing diabetes.

There are two types of diabetes. Those with type 1 diabetes don't make enough insulin to lower their blood sugar. In the past, this type was called juvenile-onset diabetes. Viruses and autoimmunity may cause it. Those with type 2 diabetes are insensitive to the insulin they have. Calorie-dense diets and a sedentary lifestyle are the major causes. In the past, this was called adult-onset diabetes; sadly, American children have become so obese that the most common type of diabetes in teenagers today is type 2.

Diabetes is not just a high-sugar disease; it is also a cardiovascular disease. People with type 2 diabetes have the same heart disease risk as those who already have heart disease. People with diabetes are not only at high risk for heart attack and stroke; they also develop narrowing of the small arteries in their kidneys, eyes, and extremities. The frequent complications of type 2 diabetes are among the many good reasons why you do not want to become obese.

Lifestyle changes are not optional for diabetic individuals; they are mandatory. Repeatedly, the Pritikin Program has been found to markedly reduce blood sugar and allow people to reduce or discontinue their medications—yet another good reason to start living the 10 Pritikin Essentials.

Metabolic Syndrome

As you have learned, abdominal obesity, high blood pressure, abnormal cholesterol, and high blood sugar often occur simultaneously in the same individual—a collection called metabolic syndrome. Metabolic syndrome is also called *dysmetabolic syndrome, syndrome X, Reaven's syndrome, insulin resistance syndrome,* and the most descriptive name, "the deadly quartet." You have metabolic syndrome if you meet at least three of the following five criteria:

- abdominal obesity (waist more than 40 inches as a man or 35 inches as a woman)
- fasting blood sugar above 100 or on diabetes medicine

- blood pressure above 130/85 or on blood pressure medicine
- HDL (good) cholesterol less than 40 as a man or 50 as a woman or on medicine to raise it
- triglycerides above 150 or taking medicine to lower it

Twenty-four percent of Americans currently have at least three of these risk factors, and therefore have metabolic syndrome. They probably already have atherosclerosis and are well on their way to having a heart attack, stroke, and diabetes. If you have metabolic syndrome, weight loss is not merely an option; it is life-saving! Again, dropping 10 to 20 pounds can make a big difference. In a recent trial, overweight individuals with mildly elevated blood sugar developed full-blown diabetes 58 percent less frequently after they lost an average of 15 pounds on a reduced-calorie, low-fat diet and exercised 150 minutes per week.

In another recently published study, three weeks of diet and exercise therapy at the Pritikin Center reversed the clinical diagnosis of metabolic syndrome in half the men studied. As pointed out in an accompanying editorial from the Washington University School of Medicine, these results were most impressive because the men did not have to wait until they had lost a lot of weight. After shedding just six to 10 pounds, they improved virtually all factors that lead to heart disease and diabetes.

HOW MUCH WATER SHOULD I DRINK EACH DAY?

If you're eating a typical American diet full of dry, salty, and highly processed foods, the oft-quoted "eight 8-ounce glasses of water a day" rule is probably necessary. But if you're eating a really healthy diet like Pritikin, full of water-rich fresh foods like fruits and vegetables, you're probably taking in plenty of water. So our advice to our Pritikin people regarding water consumption is very simple: Drink water when you're thirsty. Stop drinking when you're not.

A few other points about drinking water:

- Drink more any time your body is losing fluids, such as with exercise and during hot weather, or in dry climates, but stay away from high-calorie sports drinks.
- You can drink too much water. Some well-meaning people drink so much water that they unbalance the electrolytes in their blood, leading to a vicious cycle of more water drinking.
- Water may be the best beverage, but it does not reduce hunger by itself.
- Excessive thirst may be a sign of diabetes, hormone deficiency, or too much salt in your diet.
- Beware of anyone recommending excessive fluid intake to "cleanse your body." Your body will do just fine with a normal amount of water.
- If you have experienced kidney stones or frequent bladder infections, ask your doctor about your fluid intake, as more water may help, although cutting back on salt, meat, and certain foods high in oxalic acid, such as rhubarb and spinach, is just as important for reducing kidney stones.

CAN STRESS AND DEPRESSION MAKE ME OBESE?

Stress and depression can surely promote heart disease. The answer to whether they can cause obesity is a resounding yes and no.

Each of us responds differently to stressful circumstances. Depressions differ, as well. Some people respond to stress predominantly with adrenaline. They are the lucky "thin-nervous" types of people. Others respond with more cortisol. They are the "stressed eaters." How do you know which type you are? Since most of us Americans are stressed, just step on a scale to find out.

It's natural to seek relief when we are stressed, and for many, that relief comes in the form of comfort food. Sugar-containing foods seem to comfort us better than healthier foods, possibly by increasing brain serotonin levels. This response is common in nature. Mice, stressed by exposure to cold, stop eating their usual pellet food and switch to calorie-dense sweets and fats. But eating to relieve stress or sadness is disastrous. The resulting weight gain only makes us more depressed.

We also want emotional comfort when we are stressed. We remember the hugs that our parents gave us when we finished our plates. An ineffective response to stress is a major cause of obesity for some people. If you are a stressed eater, the only solution is to understand what is going on in your head, find ways to respond better emotionally, and snack and eat smarter even when stressed.

Depression is an extreme degree of sadness that affects activities and eating. A loss of interest in eating and many other activities is part of common depression. Unexpected weight loss can be the first evident sign of depression. Depression is a serious disorder and requires medical attention. Today, it is commonly treated with several SSRI drugs, standing for *selective serotonin reuptake inhibitors*. They increase serotonin levels in the brain, which is associated with a happier emotional state. Individual responses to these antidepressant drugs vary, but weight gain is common. If you are gaining weight on an SSRI drug, discuss the situation with your physician.

Less common than traditional depression is an atypical form, often characterized by increased sensitivity to criticism. Unlike typical depression, this form may be associated with weight gain. Individuals who experience this may be excessively self-critical, especially of their weight. This situation is self-sustaining. Unhappiness over body image leads to more depression, leading to more eating, leading to more unhappiness over body image. These people are the "unhappy eaters." It is difficult to break this cycle without psychological help, but with proper attention and care, it *can* be broken.

I do not want to leave you with the impression that all obesity is due to stress and depression. Most obesity stems from poor parenting, nutritional ignorance, excess food availability and packaging, clever fast-food marketing, poor eating habits, and inactivity. For the most part, we simply eat too much calorie-dense junk food, eat too little healthy food, and are too inactive.

CAN I DRINK ALCOHOL?

Like the meaning of life, this question has no simple answer. Alcohol is a simple sugar, but a very complex beverage. It has both beneficial and detrimental effects, even for the heart. As with many things, it comes down to moderation versus excess; like any other drug, you can ingest too little for it to have any effect, overdose on it, take it at the wrong time, or take it in a wrong combination.

Indeed, alcohol consumed in moderation does reduce atherosclerosis, which is a good thing. Middle-aged and older individuals benefit the most from alcohol because of their increasing risk of coronary heart disease. But when consumed in excess, alcohol increases blood pressure and heart rhythm disturbances and can cause heart failure. The cardiovascular benefits of alcohol must be weighed carefully against its downsides. Just to name a few, alcohol:

- Contributes to obesity
- Increases appetite
- Is a major source of violence and accidents
- Contributes to liver, pancreatic, and neurological disease
- Is associated with several cancers, including breast cancer
- Is the third leading cause of preventable premature death in the United States (100,000 Americans die each year from alcohol-associated diseases and trauma)
- Creates habituation in 10 percent of its frequent users

Assuming you enjoy drinking, Pritikin recommends that men should limit their intake to seven drinks per week and women to four drinks per week, to avoid the calories and serious side effects. You might be surprised, though, to find out just how much "one drink" actually is. One drink is defined as:

- 12 ounces of beer
- four to five ounces of wine (⅙ bottle)
- 1½ ounces of whiskey (1 jigger)

All of these beverage amounts supply about ½ ounce of pure alcohol. While most people understand that a 12-ounce can or bottle of beer is one drink, many are surprised to learn that a jigger of whiskey is 1 drink and that a wine bottle contains five to six drinks, almost the same as a six-pack of beer. The standard 24-ounce wine bottle was the original "super-size" portion.

Is red wine the best choice?

To answer this question, we need to know how alcohol reduces heart disease. The best explanation is that alcohol increases HDL (good) cholesterol. On average, HDL cholesterol increases about 5 to 10 percent if you have one drink per day. That increase is equivalent to jogging about five to ten miles per week (no, this does *not* mean you can replace exercise with a good cabernet). And, ultimately, when it comes to the variable amount alcohol raises your HDL (good) cholesterol, it does not matter whether you choose to drink wine, beer, or whiskey. The net results are generally the same.

But what about all the hoopla about the red wine–drinking French and their heart health? You may have heard about resveratrol—the anti-aging substance in red wine. What you didn't hear is that the amount tested required drinking 100 bottles of red wine per day. The French may indeed have less heart disease, but they also are less inclined to list it on death certificates in circumstances where it probably was the cause. And, they don't live significantly longer than Americans do.

There is no advantage of red wine over other beverages shown in American studies. In the largest American trial done by the Kaiser HMO, almost 129,000 Californians were followed for 13 years according to their alcohol consumption. Moderate drinkers experienced 30 percent fewer deaths, mostly due to a reduction in heart disease. *The type of alco-*

hol consumed made absolutely no difference. As a caution, though, it's worth noting here that the women in that study who drank heavily had especially high mortality rates. I choose to emphasize the Californian data over that from Europe since Californians are much more like Americans.

Although what kind of alcohol you drink makes little difference, your drinking pattern does matter. Drink in moderation regularly rather than saving it up for holidays and weekends. Heavy binge drinking does not reduce heart disease. And if you drink, of course, please drink responsibly!

WHAT NON-FOOD FACTORS HELP WEIGHT LOSS?

Besides a good diet and exercise, are there methods that can help us lose weight effectively? There has been a lot of hype and confusion in recent years about what is safe and what isn't. Here are the facts.

Nonprescription Weight-Loss Aids

Ephedrine and *ephedra* are brain and heart stimulants in the same amphetamine family. Both suppress appetite to some degree. They were sold in hundreds of weight-loss preparations until recently, often in combination with caffeine. None of these preparations met the government standards for safety and efficacy required of pharmaceuticals. Moreover, these appetite-suppressing stimulants do not work well. Studies have found that they decrease weight by about two pounds over three to six months. That is not much compared with their downside.

Taken in excess, these stimulants cause fast heart rhythms, strokes, heart attacks, and sudden death. I have taken care of two young women that suffered heart attacks probably due to these weight-loss stimulants. Please do not try to obtain these now-banned ephedra diet products. The potent hunger-suppressing combination stimulant "fen-phen" causes serious heart valve problems and lethal high blood pressure in the lungs. Thankfully, it has been removed from the market.

Prescription Weight-Loss Drugs

Sibutramine (marketed under the trade name Meridia) is a prescription appetite suppressant. Volunteers taking this drug lost about 10 more pounds over six months while dieting than those taking a placebo. Discuss with your physician whether this drug is right for you.

Another prescription and newly over-the-counter drug, orlistat (marketed under the trade names Xenical and Alli), blocks fat absorption by inactivating the intestinal enzyme that digests it. Some of the fat you eat will just pass through your digestive tract. In a recent six-month study, it was shown that orlistat increased weight loss by about eight pounds. The drug's downside is that it blocks the absorption of good and essential fats and fat-soluble vitamins. Also, severe or uncontrollable diarrhea can occur if you eat too much fat while taking the drug. It is a great teaching tool to help you avoid eating a lot of fat; you will not eat a high-fat meal on orlistat more than once. Discuss orlistat with your physician before choosing this option.

Gastric Bypass

The term *morbidly obese* applies to individuals whose weight is threatening their lives. Morbidly obese people generally have difficulty losing much weight through diet and walking, since they have long escaped their normal regulatory mechanisms. (Many, though, have lost considerable weight on the Pritikin Program, so serious diet and exercise regimens should always be considered prior to surgical options.) If they cannot lose weight, gastric bypass surgery in its various forms is an option, since they are in danger of dying.

Gastric bypass surgery generally works well. Most morbidly obese individuals lose considerable pounds after this surgery, although the weight can return. In morbidly obese patients, gastric bypass surgery reduces high blood pressure, diabetes, and cardiovascular disease. On the downside, vomiting, diarrhea, and nutrient absorption problems may result, as well as the possibility of surgical complications.

Morbidly obese individuals should carefully discuss the various types of gastric bypass surgery with a knowledgeable physician. It may save their life.

Upcoming Treatments

A drug called rimonabant, which blocks natural pleasure receptors, is currently under investigation. Obese people in a recent study lost about 12 pounds on rimonabant in a year. It also lowers cholesterol and preferentially reduces abdominal obesity, the most dangerous kind. However, emotional depression is a side effect, so much so that the FDA denied the approval of rimonabant for weight loss because its use was associated with increased suicidal tendencies.

Another interesting approach uses a small pacemaker to electrically stimulate the stomach, tricking your brain into thinking that you are full. Surgery is required to implant the pacemaker, but initial results with this approach are promising. Of course, a big green salad or bean- and veggie-rich soup at the start of a meal does just about the same and is a whole lot cheaper.

HOW CAN WE IMPROVE AMERICA'S LIFESTYLE?

You have responsibility for your own lifestyle and health, but you also have additional responsibilities. You are responsible for your children, your other family members, your community, and for this great nation. Heart disease is the canary in the mine of how we live. If we have a lot of heart disease, we have neither a happy nor a healthy lifestyle.

Our Children

Appropriately, let's start with our children. We know that lifestyle patterns are established early in life—smoking, diet, and physical activity are good examples. More important is the fact that atherosclerosis starts in children. Children rarely have heart attacks, but they are certainly developing the atherosclerosis that will cause future heart disease. Sixty percent of 22-year-old Americans dying accidentally already have coronary artery disease at autopsy. Five to ten percent of 22-year-olds have at least 50 percent blockage of a coronary artery. The foundation of heart disease prevention starts with our children.

We need to encourage weight loss in children without hurting their self-image. To achieve this goal, it is up to every one of us as adults to become good role models of healthy lifestyles and appropriate weight. Minimize the time your children spend in front of the television; this is an important feature for controlling the potential for obesity. The time children spend watching television or playing electronic games can be so much better spent being physically active or mentally creative.

Eat meals with your children. Teach them to enjoy the same meals: above two years of age, children can and should eat adult food. That means eating salads, soups, fruits, and vegetables. Serve only appropriately small portions of calorie-dense food, such as peanut butter and jelly sandwiches. Do not prepare all-in-one packaged meals; they are generally loaded with fat, sugar, and salt. If you have the time, cook from scratch. At the very least, stay far away from fast-food establishments. A "Happy Meal" does not make for a happy heart later in life.

Keep the junk food out of your home. Stock up on fresh fruits and vegetables. Make fruit the preferred dessert and reward. Buy skim milk or flavored soymilk and keep cold water in the refrigerator. If you must serve sodas, make them diet sodas. Make healthy lunches for your children to take to school, at least through elementary school. Demand that your children's school cafeteria prepare healthy food. Above all, do not demand that your children finish the food on their plates. They will eat when they get hungry and stop when they are filled.

Encourage your children to be physically active and take part in sports. Walking and bicycling should be lifelong activities. Get children accustomed to using their feet to get somewhere. Use recreational facilities if there aren't sidewalks or bike lanes. Encourage lifelong competitive sports, such as tennis and soccer, or basketball in the driveway. Don't emphasize sports that require bulk. People rarely play such sports all their life, but they can remain bulked up forever. Stress the participation, not the winning. Attend your children's sporting events. Be in touch with your children. Carefully observe how they interact with others at play. It's far more important than whether their team wins.

Do everything you can to prevent your children from starting smoking. Start by being a nonsmoker yourself. Allow them to rebel in less destructive ways. If your children can get to their early twenties as nonsmokers, their intelligence and self-esteem are likely to develop to the point that they have a good chance of never starting. Do not think that it is okay for them to "experiment" with smoking. Nicotine addiction occurs faster in children than in adults. Some studies show that addiction begins with one pack of cigarettes. If your children start smoking, do everything you can to exorcise them of this habit. It is not a passing fad. This awful habit will cost them 10 percent of their life.

Insist that your children get the best and the most education. Education is not only important for their future, it is important for their health. As educational level increases, heart diseases and several other illnesses decrease. In this country, obesity, diabetes, hypertension, kidney disease, heart disease, and cancer are more common among less educated people. Knowledge is not only wealth; it is health. Education lessens risk factors for heart disease and improves the outcome of those who get heart disease. In matters of lifestyle, ignorance is not bliss. The button on my white coat says, "It's too bad that ignorance isn't painful."

Make sure that your children get regular medical care. We may have the most sophisticated medical technology in this country, but we rank with Honduras in standards of basic medical care, such as immunization and infant mortality. Follow weight and blood pressure carefully in children. Your cuddly, chubby kid may be seriously overweight when viewed through the objective eyes of your pediatrician. Cholesterol should be measured in children if either parent has high cholesterol or heart disease.

Teach your children friendship and love, the key ingredients in emotional nourishment. Know their friends. Encourage their friendships with other children of whom you approve. Teach them how to focus on the good qualities and achievements of their friends. You need to take as much credit for their hatred and prejudice as for their good looks and intelligence. Teach them loyalty, responsibility, discipline, and respect. But let them be kids. Let them get dirty. Let them goof off some of the time. Above all, give them unconditional love.

Develop community and school-based health programs for children. Our friend Dr. Kim Eagle helped to start a middle-school program in Ann Arbor, Michigan. The program teaches healthy eating, promotes physical fitness, and encourages school administrators to offer better food choices. Why? Thirty-two percent of the Ann Arbor kids were overweight, 10 percent already had high cholesterol, and 9 percent already had high blood pressure. Another friend, Florida school superintendent Rudy Crew, has promised to do the same, and is meeting with our dieticians who teach the Pritikin Family Program, a program in healthy living for kids and parents held every summer at Pritikin. We cannot call ourselves a great country if we continue to sell out our children.

The really good news is that the benefits our children derive from healthy habits can happen quickly and profoundly. In research published in 2007 in the journal *Atherosclerosis* on overweight kids attending the Pritikin Family Program, UCLA scientists found that in just two weeks, the kids:

- Lowered total cholesterol on average 23 percent
- Decreased LDL (bad) cholesterol 25 percent
- Shed 9 pounds

- Lowered triglyceride fats 39 percent
- Reduced key markers of inflammation, including C-reactive protein and oxidative stress
- Increased the body's production of beneficial nitric oxide

Our Spouses

Remember, emotional connection is a key component of happiness and health. Enjoy and provide for each other. There will be ups and downs, but always fight cleanly. You can argue while demonstrating affection and commitment. Provide each other with what you really need, namely time, love, friendship, and sex, as well as the material needs. Figure out what you really do need and do not waste time going after what you don't need. You can change some traits through affection, but you can never change each other by demand. Learn to accept and not criticize your spouse's faults that you cannot change.

Interpret your spouse's intentions and qualities under the most favorable light. He or she is yours, one hopes more for better than for worse. Remember, friendship, affection, and love start with a favorable perception. Ask yourself whether you would like to be married to someone like yourself. If the answer is no, adjust accordingly! Our country's almost 50 percent divorce rate speaks volumes about our self-centered inflexibility. Divorce is not only expensive; it ranks with the death of a loved one as a leading emotional factor for heart attacks. Head off your spouse's obesity, inactivity, poor diet, alcoholism, and medical procrastination before they become ingrained in his or her lifestyle.

Our Country

Here are our 10 Pritikin prescriptions for a better American lifestyle:

1. We need to acknowledge that America has a lifestyle problem. Obesity, lousy diet, physical inactivity, and emotional malnutrition are vitally important issues. The hundreds of billions of

health-care dollars we spend fixing the consequences of our lifestyle means a loss in economic vitality. I recently spoke with the commander of a naval base involved in military recruiting. One of the biggest obstacles to recruiting is that many young people simply cannot pass the fitness requirements. Lifestyle is an issue of national security. We need to begin a national dialogue on lifestyle.

2. Start taxing sugar-containing beverages. Every 12-ounce sugar-containing beverage increases health-care costs by about 17 cents. Producers and consumers should pay for the health-care costs they incur. Banning sugary drinks would not be popular, but it would cure a good chunk of obesity in America within five years.

3. Tax junk food. Ban its advertisement on children's television. Junk food is not difficult to identify. It's like obscenity; you cannot define it, but you know it when you see it.

4. Label all sizes of packaged foods meant for one person with their total calories, not calories per portion. People seldom look at how many portions they contain. The total calorie content has recently been added to the per-portion calories. That is a start, but drop the per-portion information on containers meant for one person. For example, up to 24 ounces of a beverage is really meant for one person. Of course, 24 ounces is a ridiculous portion, but that is what some of us consume. Require chain restaurants to list calories and nutrients as New York City recently has.

5. Encourage walking and bicycling. It's cheap, nonpolluting, healthful, and enjoyable. Almost every other civilized country pays much more than us for gas. America subsidizes its petroleum industry. Whatever we are paying at the pump, we need to add the medical cost of inactivity and the human and financial burden of Middle East military maneuvers. Only in America do people driving SUVs demand cheaper gas. Have we become so literally and figuratively fat that we can no longer squeeze into

smaller cars? Do not vote for politicians who don't drive a hybrid or smaller car. They are hypocrites, not statesmen.

6. Get all children involved in sports programs at or after school. Give tax breaks for exercise facilities at work. Sidewalks and bike paths also help.

7. Encourage working together and community service in schools. Teamwork is more than sweating at an athletic event together. Our children need to learn responsibility for others. Social responsibility and connectedness is good for physical and mental health.

8. Pay doctors more for preventive care and less for complex treatments. You will get what you pay for. We perform expensive heart angioplasties and bypass operations two to 10 times more frequently than other advanced countries. Why? Because we pay physicians much more for doing expensive procedures than for educating patients about healthy living. Preventing disease in the first place makes the most sense, especially if we use lifestyle changes.

9. Teach preventive medicine in schools and make the national standards for treating cholesterol, high blood pressure, and diabetes stricter. Three-quarters of individuals suffering a heart attack would not qualify for cholesterol-lowering measures the day before by the current guidelines. Using intensive preventive care, we can eliminate at least half of the heart attacks and strokes that occur with existing routine care. That is a proven benefit.

10. Insure health care for all Americans, emphasizing lifestyle changes. Stratify health-care insurance premiums by modifiable risk factors, such as weight, blood pressure, and cholesterol. Reduce premiums when risk factors improve. We pay more for life insurance the older we get because we are more likely to need it. A poor lifestyle similarly increases medical-care costs. When we Americans finally realize that a poor lifestyle is costly, as well as unhealthy and depressing, we will

change to a healthier and happier one. We will change to the Pritikin Program.

MARGARET'S LAST VISIT

I got a postcard from Cancún in February on a cold day in Annapolis. It simply said: "Thanks, Margaret."

I saw Margaret for the last time in May, almost a year to the day I first saw her. She weighed in at 136 pounds, just four pounds short of her goal. She had lost 36 pounds and her waist measured 32 inches. Her blood pressure was 126 over 78, her LDL (bad) cholesterol was 97, and her HDL (good) cholesterol was 56. Margaret's outdoor tennis league had just started, and she was confident that she would reach her weight goal within a month or two.

I asked her what she has learned about lifestyle during the past year. She told me that she was spending less time in the office and more at activities that she really enjoyed, such as tennis. Her job had not suffered. In fact, she had received a minor promotion. She had learned to eat tastier, more filling food, while losing weight. The realization that satisfying food was no longer her enemy was a welcome surprise.

She and her husband had gotten into the habit of eating leisurely, larger, but less calorie-dense dinners after walking their dog. They had discovered that good food was better than bad TV. They always delayed their dessert for at least an hour after dinner, only to find that a relatively small portion was very satisfying by then. Margaret and her husband usually treated themselves to a small bowl of low-fat chocolate ice cream for dessert, along with a second cup of decaf coffee. I smiled and confessed that my wife and I do the same, almost every night.

Margaret then told me what I really wanted to hear. She was indeed happier. She liked herself better and she was getting along well at the office, with her friends, and in her marriage. Her husband told her that he really liked how she looked in a bathing suit, which made her feel great. (I told her that we men are all the same. She agreed on that!) On her way out of the office, she told me that she had come to understand that a "happier and healthier lifestyle was always there for the taking." I asked if I could quote her on that.

10 Resistance Exercises for Losing Fat and Building Muscle

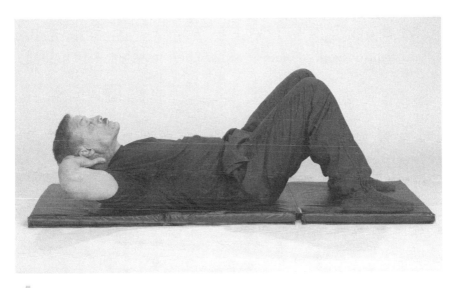

1. ABDOMINAL CRUNCH (abdominals)

- Lie on exercise mat, keeping your head and neck in line with your spine.

Put your hands in one of the following three positions: 1) hands reaching toward knees, 2) hands placed across chest, or 3) hands behind and supporting head. Elevate your shoulders and upper back toward your knees. Keep your lower back and middle back on mat. Repeat 8 to 15 times for 1 to 3 sets.

2. **OBLIQUE CRUNCH** (obliques)

- Lie on exercise mat, keeping your head and neck in line with spine.
- Place your right hand behind your head to support the head. Place your left arm perpendicular to the left side of your body and place your left ankle on your right knee.
- Lift your right shoulder blade off the mat toward the ceiling, slightly angling toward your left knee. Repeat 8 to 15 times on each side for 1 to 3 sets.

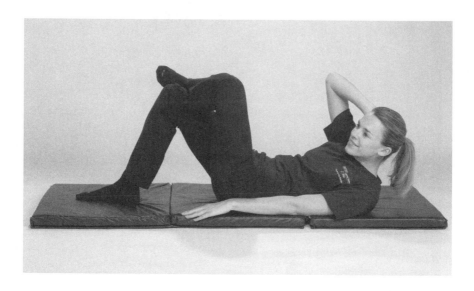

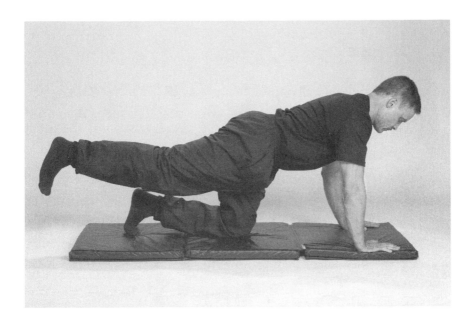

3. **HIP EXTENSION ON ALL FOURS** (low back, hamstrings, and gluteals)

- On exercise mat, start on all fours with your hands placed directly under your shoulders. (If you have shoulder pain, support yourself with your elbows instead of your hands.) Your knees should be directly under hips.
- Extend your right leg backward, approximately parallel to floor, with the knee slightly bent, and hold for a 2-second count. Be careful not to arch your neck or back. Repeat 8 to 15 times with each leg for 1 to 3 sets.

NOTE: *If you have lower back concerns, proceed with caution or avoid this exercise.*

4. **SQUAT** (quadriceps, gluteals, and hamstrings)

- Choose dumbbells and then place your hands (holding the weights) at your sides. Stand with your feet wider than your shoulders. Slightly bend your knees.
- To begin repetition, slowly lower yourself toward the floor (as if you were squatting) until your thighs are almost parallel to the ground.
- Return to starting position (keeping a slight bend in your knees). Remember to keep your back straight and your shoulders back at all times. Repeat 8 to 15 times for 1 to 3 sets.

NOTE: *If you have knee concerns, proceed with caution or avoid this exercise.*

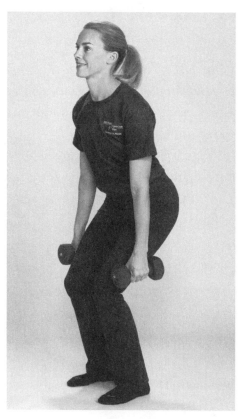

5. CALF RAISE (calves)

- Choose dumbbells and then place your hands (holding the weights) at your sides.
- Next, stand with your feet wider than your shoulders. Straighten your knees and rise onto the balls of your feet, raising your heels off the floor.
- Return to the starting position by slowly lowering your heels to the floor. Repeat 8 to 15 times for 1 to 3 sets.

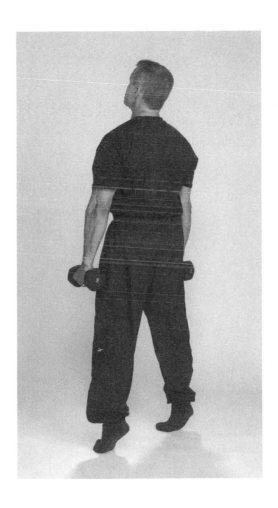

6. CHEST PRESS (chest, triceps, and shoulders)

- Lie on exercise bench with a dumbbell in each hand, elbows bent (in a position that is similar to pushing a grocery cart).
- Extend your arms up slowly toward ceiling, until they're straight.
- Lower slowly to starting position. Repeat 8 to 15 times for 1 to 3 sets.

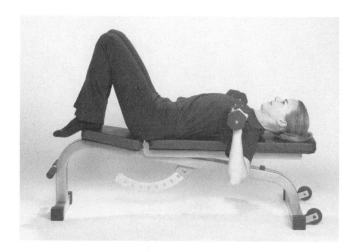

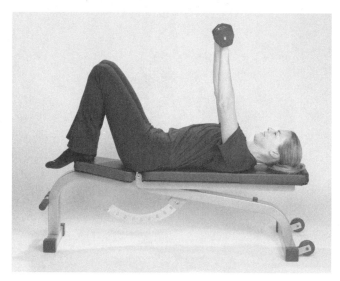

7. ONE-ARM ROW (upper/middle back, shoulders, and biceps)

- Place your right hand and right knee on exercise bench and extend your left foot out to the side, standing on it for balance.
- Next, pick up a dumbbell with your left hand, letting your left arm extend below your left shoulder.
- To begin repetition, slowly lift the weight up so that in the finished position the dumbbell is at the left side of your torso, just in front of the hip. Lower the weight back down to the starting position. Repeat 8 to 15 times with each arm for 1 to 3 sets.

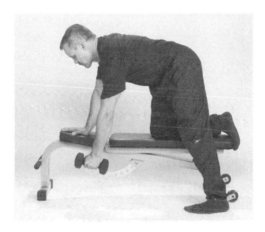

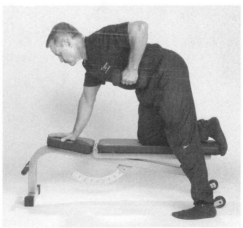

8. **LATERAL RAISE** (shoulders)

- Start with your arms resting at your sides and holding a dumb-bell in each hand.
- Slowly raise your arms to shoulder height with elbows slightly bent. Make sure palms are facing down.
- Slowly lower the arms back down to your sides. Repeat 8 to 15 times for 1 to 3 sets.

NOTE: *If you have shoulder or neck concerns, proceed with caution or avoid this exercise.*

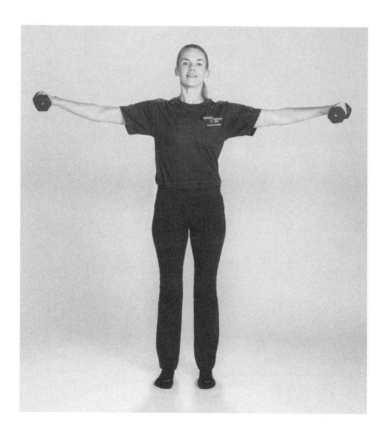

9. **BICEP CURL** (biceps)

- Stand with knees slightly bent, feet shoulder-width apart, holding a dumbbell in each hand. Make sure your arms are resting at your sides and your palms are facing in front of you.
- Keeping your elbows slightly bent and against your sides, curl both hands toward your shoulders. Lower your hands to starting position. Repeat 8 to 15 times for 1 to 3 sets.

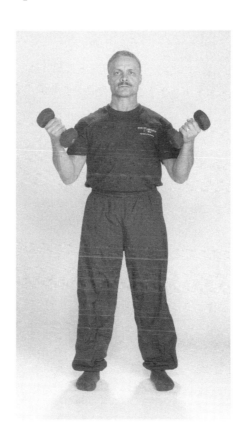

10. ONE-ARM TRICEP KICKBACK (triceps)

- Stand next to exercise bench and place your right knee and right hand on bench for support.
- Pick up a weight with your left hand and bring your left elbow up so that your upper arm is parallel to the ground and your hand holding the dumbbell is hanging down below your elbow. This is your starting position.
- Extend your left arm backward, straightening it. Lower slowly to starting position. Repeat for 8 to 15 times with each arm for 1 to 3 sets.

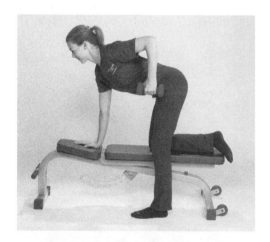

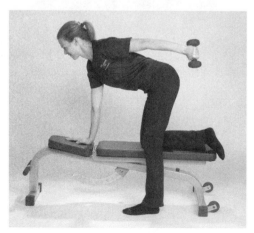

Full-Body Stretching Routine

1. STANDING NECK CLOCK STRETCH

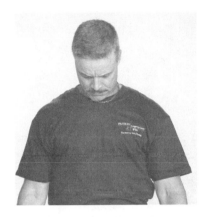

a. Drop your chin to your chest and hold for 10 to 30 seconds.

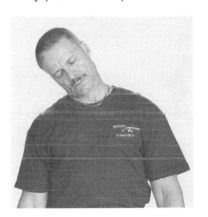
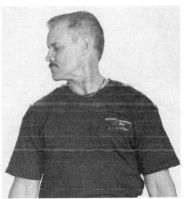

b. Drop your right ear to your right shoulder and hold for 10 to 30 seconds.

c. Look over your right shoulder and hold for 10 to 30 seconds.

d. Repeat b and c for left side of body.

CAUTION: *Do not tilt your head back. This may add unnecessary pressure to your neck.*

2. STANDING SHOULDER STRETCH

- Grasp your right arm just behind your elbow with your left hand and gently pull the arm across your chest until a stretch is felt in the right shoulder.
- Hold for 10 to 30 seconds.
- Repeat with the other arm.

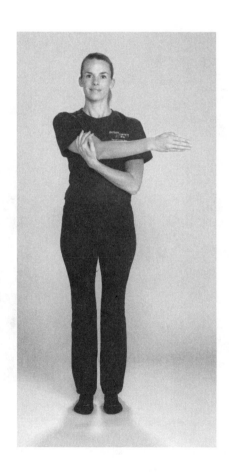

3. STANDING TRICEP STRETCH

- Place your right hand on your right shoulder blade. With your left hand, gently grasp your right elbow and press your right elbow straight up toward your head until you feel the stretch in the back of your arm.
- Hold for 10 to 30 seconds.
- Repeat with the other arm.

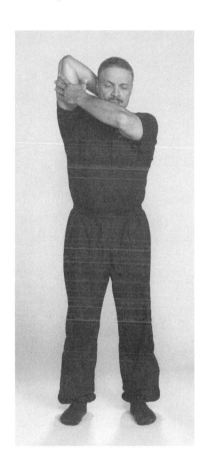 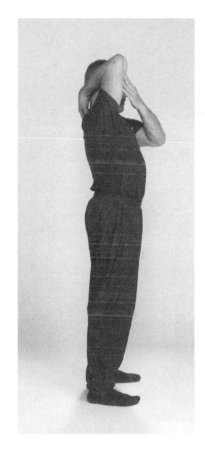

4. STANDING UPPER BACK STRETCH

- Place both hands together out in front of your chest. Extend your arms and push your palms forward in front of you. Lower your chin to your chest. Round your shoulder blades so you feel the stretch in the upper back.
- Hold for 10 to 30 seconds.

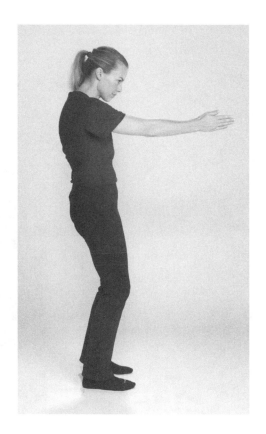

5. STANDING CHEST STRETCH

- Open up your arms with your thumbs up. Squeeze your shoulder blades together while reaching arms behind you to feel the stretch in your chest.
- Hold for 10 to 30 seconds.

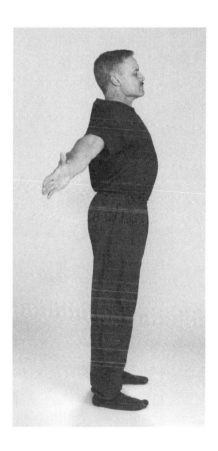

6. STANDING CALF STRETCH

- Begin by standing in front of an unmovable object, such as a table or wall. Place your hands on the object at shoulder width.
- Place your right foot forward with knee bent. Keep the left leg straight and press the left heel to the floor. Feel the stretch on the lower portion of the left leg.
- Hold for 10 to 30 seconds.
- Repeat with the other leg.

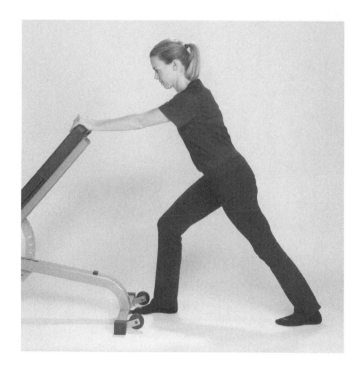

7. STANDING ACHILLES TENDON STRETCH

- Begin by standing in front of an unmovable object, such as a table or wall. Place your hands on the unmovable object at shoulder width.
- Place your right foot forward, left foot back. Bend both knees slightly, keeping your heels on the ground. Feel the stretch near the left heel. Hold for 10 to 30 seconds.
- Repeat with the other leg.

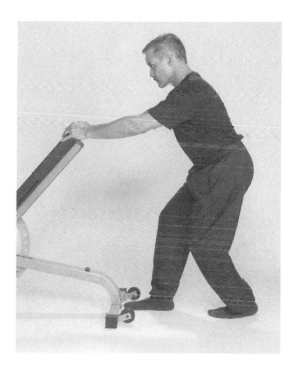

8. STANDING HAMSTRING STRETCH

- Slightly bend your left leg and place your right foot on a low-to-high support in front of you.
- Place your hands on top of your right thigh and bend forward from the hips until you feel a stretch along the back of the right thigh. Hold for 10 to 30 seconds.
- Repeat with the other leg.

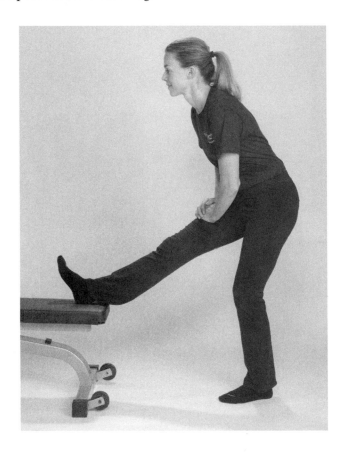

9. STANDING QUADRICEP STRETCH

- Slightly bend your left leg and bring your right leg up behind you. Grasp your ankle with your right hand. If you are unable to comfortably reach your ankle, grab the back of your sock or heel of your shoe, or loop a towel or stretching strap around your ankle. Gently pull the right ankle back toward the hip joint.
- To protect the knee, your heel should not touch your buttocks. Feel the stretch along the front of the right thigh. Hold for 10 to 30 seconds.
- Repeat with the other leg.

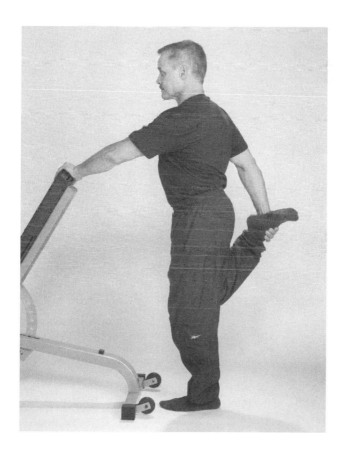

10. SEATED TORSO STRETCH

- Sit on the floor and place your right hand on floor beside your hip for support. Reach your left arm over head as you tilt your torso toward the right. Keep your buttocks on the ground and avoid bending forward or backward.
- Feel the stretch along the left side of the torso. Hold for 10 to 30 seconds.
- Repeat on the other side.

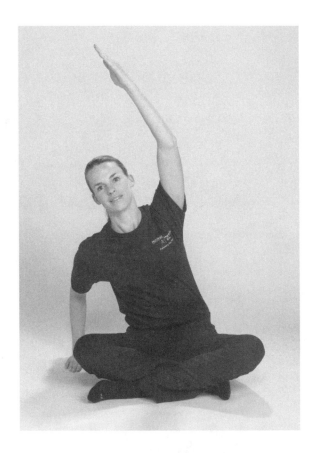

11. SEATED GROIN STRETCH

- While seated on the floor, bend your knees and place the soles of your feet together.
- Grasp your ankles and relax the knees toward the floor without using your elbows to put pressure on your knees. Feel the stretch along the inner thigh of both legs. Hold for 10 to 30 seconds.

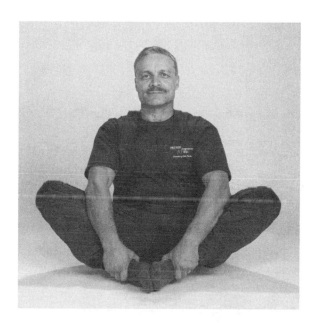

12. SEATED HAMSTRING STRETCH

- While seated on the floor, straighten your right leg. With your left knee bent, place the sole of your left foot on the inside of your right leg.
- Place your hands on floor behind your hips and gently press your torso forward directly over the right leg, keeping your back straight. Feel the stretch along the back of the right leg and lower back. Hold for 10 to 30 seconds.
- Repeat with the other leg.

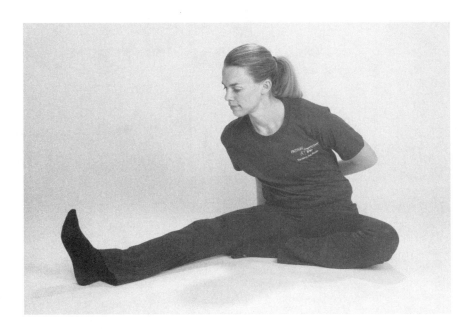

13. SUPINE QUADRICEP STRETCH

- Lying on your left side, grasp your right ankle with your right hand. If you are unable to comfortably reach your ankle, grab the back of your sock or heel of your shoe, or loop a towel or stretching strap around your ankle. Gently pull the ankle back toward the hip joint.
- To protect your knee, your heel should not touch your buttocks. Feel the stretch along the front of the right thigh. Hold for 10 to 30 seconds.
- Repeat with the other leg.

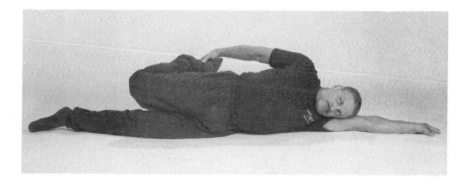

14. SUPINE GLUTEAL AND LOWER BACK STRETCH

- Lie on your back, knees bent and feet flat on the floor. Place both hands behind right thigh. If you are unable to comfortably reach behind the leg, loop a towel or stretching strap around the back of your thigh.
- Gently pull your leg as close to your chest as possible, feeling the stretch on the right side of the gluteal and lower back. To protect your back, keep the left leg bent with your foot on the floor. Hold for 10 to 30 seconds.
- Repeat with the other leg.

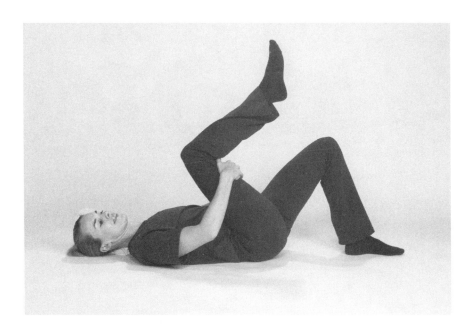

15. SUPINE HAMSTRING STRETCH

- Lie on your back, knees bent and feet flat on the floor. Extend your right leg up, keeping the leg as straight as possible.
- Place both hands behind the back of your right leg and gently pull to feel the stretch along the back of your right thigh. If you are unable to comfortably pull the leg with your hands, loop a towel or stretching strap around the back of your leg or arch of your foot. Hold for 10 to 30 seconds.
- Repeat with the other leg.

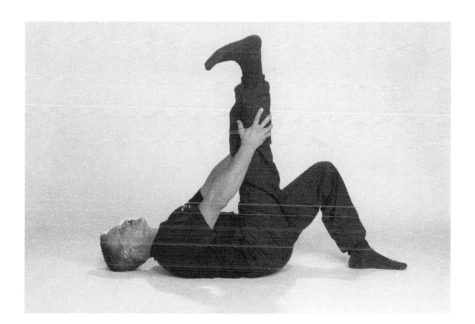

16. MAD CAT UPPER BACK STRETCH

- Begin on your hands and knees, with your hands directly under your shoulders and shoulder width apart, and your knees directly under your hips and hip width apart.
- Simultaneously, drop your chin to your chest, pull your stomach toward your spine, and arch your back up like a mad cat. Feel the stretch in your upper back.
- Hold for 10 to 30 seconds.

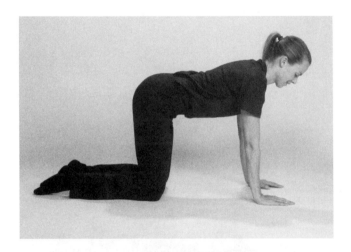

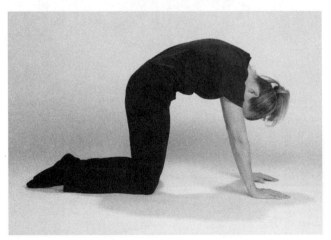

Daily Nutrition Analysis with Weekly Average—Week 1

Nutrient	Day 1	Day 2	Day 3	Day 4	Day 5	Day 6	Day 7	Week 1 Averages	IOM* Recommendations
Calories	1638	1839	1613	1672	1599	1632	1630	1660	—
Calorie Density (cal/lb)	245	237	242	272	366	289	259	273	—
% Protein	18	23	21	18	20	20	21	20	10–35%
% Carbohydrate	66	63	65	62	65	64	69	65	45–65%
Total Fat (g)	29	29	25	38	26	29	18	28	—
% Fat	16	14	14	20	15	16	10	15	< 35%
Saturated Fat (g)	4	6	4	4	6	5	3	4.6	—
% Saturated Fat	2	3	2	2	3	2	2	2.3	as low as possible
Omega-3 (g)	3	1	1	4	2	3	1	2.1	—
Omega-6 (g)	6	4	5	14	8	6	3	6.6	—
Omega-6:Omega-3 Ratio	2 to 1	4 to 1	5 to 1	3.5 to 1	4 to 1	2 to 1	3 to 1	3.4 to 1	—
Cholesterol (mg)	72	44	46	49	54	113	76	65	as low as possible
Dietary Fiber (g)	41	84	39	51	50	50	49	52	> 25g
Sodium (mg)	1283	1329	1426	1339	1474	1533	1417	1400	1200–1500mg

*Institute of Medicine, Dietary Reference Intakes www.iom.edu

Daily Nutrition Analysis with Weekly Average—Week 2

Nutrient	Day 8	Day 9	Day 10	Day 11	Day 12	Day 13	Day 14	Week 2 Averages	IOM* Recommendations
Calories	1611	1623	1656	1617	1602	1612	1595	1617	—
Calorie Density (cal/lb)	299	301	278	290	275	251	296	284	—
% Protein	19	21	21	21	21	20	19	20	10–35%
% Carbohydrate	66	62	66	68	64	67	64	65	45–65%
Total Fat (g)	26	30	24	19	26	23	30	25	—
% Fat	15	17	13	11	15	13	17	14	<35%
Saturated Fat (g)	4	6	5	3	3	3	3	3.9	—
% Saturated Fat	2	3	3	2	2	2	2	2.3	as low as possible
Omega-3 (g)	1	4	1	3	2	1	3	2.1	—
Omega-6 (g)	4	6	4	5	9	3	11	6.0	—
Omega-6:Omega-3 Ratio	4 to 1	1.5 to 1	4 to 1	1.7 to 1	4.5 to 1	3 to 1	3.7 to 1	3.2 to 1	—
Cholesterol (mg)	24	63	96	72	97	17	39	58	as low as possible
Dietary Fiber (g)	39	44	47	43	43	52	39	44	> 25g
Sodium (mg)	1470	1228	1482	1472	1511	1407	1330	1414	1200–1500mg

*Institute of Medicine, Dietary Reference Intakes www.iom.edu

Index

Index of Recipes